KETO BREAD:

150 low carb recipes for your weight loss goals including desserts, gluten-free and everything you need to know about baking and ketogenic diet in one cookbook.

KIMBERLY MADISON

TABLE OF CONTENTS

Introduction

Those who have been struggling with weight loss and trying to keep them off but couldn't would understand that the visceral fat are the hardest to lose. But with the ketogenic diet, this is possible.

To get the leaner and fitter physique, this diet teaches the body on how to turn it into usable energy and convert stored fat thereby speeding up weight loss. For first time followers of the ketogenic diet, it should be noted that carbohydrates found in starchy vegetables, grains, and those in other fruits are not advised to be consumed. Instead, take more of meat, dairy products, seeds, and nuts.

Nowadays people follow various diets to improve their health and lose weight. The ketogenic paleo diet is one of the most popular diets amongst them. It is actually a combination of the keto and paleo diets.

This diet is also known as the caveman's diet. The underlying principle for this diet is that optimal health can be promoted by eating the foods that were partaken by the early man.

According to this diet, the modern systems of producing and processing food are harmful for human health. So you can support the natural biological functioning of the body and improve digestion and overall health if you imitate the eating habits of the paleolithic people who were hunter-gatherers.

Paleo eliminates legumes, grains, most of the dairy sources, and processed sugar. The foods that are permitted in this diet include fish and meat, eggs, seeds and nuts, vegetables, fruits, and selected oils and fats such as olive oil, coconut oil, ghee, butter, tallow, lard and avocado oil. Besides this, sweeteners that are minimally processed like maple syrup, raw stevia, coconut sugar, and raw honey are allowed.

Mostly, the body's tissues prefer to get energy from the glucose derived from carbohydrates. But there is a metabolic state known as ketosis when the body utilizes the calories gained from fat rather than that derived from carbs to get the energy for carrying out the normal functions.

The goal of the ketogenic or keto diet is to induce this state by adjusting the macronutrients, namely fat, protein, and carbohydrates.

The physiological state that is called ketosis makes it possible for the body to lose more fats. You will learn more about ketosis as you go through the book. This diet also prevents the warning signs of type ii diabetes and delays the onset of alzheimer's disease. If you are undergoing ketosis, you will notice that you don't feel hungry in between meals and don't crave for sweets and fatty food.

Maintaining a low carbohydrate diet will keep all lifestyle diseases and their complications at bay. This also lessens the risk of stroke and other cardiovascular diseases.

Any of these adversities can result in bread that is hard, tough. Fortunately, using a bread machine makes bread almost foolproof. You don't have to care about how much dough to knead or whether the bread dough will rise or not. The machine does all of this for you. Now that you know the benefits of a bread machine, it's time to choose one that suits you.

If you want to know more about this diet and the many recipes that you can make, go through the pages of this book and consider this your first step towards welcoming the new you that your future self will thank you for.

Thanks again for downloading this book. I hope you enjoy it!

Chapter 1. Everything You Need To Know About The Ketogenic Diet

The ketogenic diet has become popular when it proved effective as means to lose stubborn body fat. It was first designed to control the effects of epilepsy in children. The very principle of this diet is ketosis or the process where the body burns off stored fats.

The body undergoes the state of ketosis the moment glucose from carbohydrates are strictly lessened or totally removed from one's diet. We all know that glucose is the chief fuel of the brain. When you're in ketosis, your brain pushes the pancreas but, in such circumstances,, the brain rewires and pushes the pancreas to make high amounts of ketone bodies – these are water soluble molecules that breaks down fat in the adipose tissues. The fat converted are absorbed by the brain and becomes the body's energy source.

So, when does ketosis happens? It happens after 2 to 7 days of steady and regular caloric deprivation or what they call the low-carbohydrate consumption. By that time, the human brain is fast burning lipids, converting into free fatty acids, which are processed as an energy fuel. In order to achieve effective weight loss and lifelong health, ketosis should be continued for as long as possible or until you have achieved your desired weight goal. Of course, it would be better if this becomes part of your lifestyle. Note however, that any carbohydrate or sugar intake in the duration of the diet could mean going back to step one. That simply means no cheating on this diet.

Computing your fat intake is simple. All you have to do is get your prescribed number of calories for each day and multiply by 0.70. The required calories should be between 1,500 to 2,000 calories per day. Divide the result by 9 and you'll get the recommended grams of fat per day. Why divide the result by 9, you might ask? It is because fat contains 9 grams of calories.

Take a look at this sample computation:

1, 500 calories x 0.70 = 1,050 – 9 = 116 grams of fat per day

The following are food list that you can include in your diet:

Your ketogenic diet should include 70% good, healthy fats such as butter, avocado oil, cocoa butter, coconut butter, coconut oil, olive oil, extra virgin olive oil, fish oil from salmon or tuna among others, sesame oil, lard, walnut oil, palm oil, and flax oil.

Some of the best sources of healthy fats include:

✓ avocadoes – 82.5% fat

✓ bacon – 69.5% fat

✓ butter – 100% fat

✓ cheddar cheese – 74% fat

✓ chicken eggs – 61% fat

✓ coconut flesh/meat – 88% fat

✓ coconut oil – 100% fat

✓ cream cheese – 88.5% fat

✓ sour cream – 88.5% fat

✓ unsweetened dark chocolate – 65% fat

✓ ground beef – 59.5% fat

Fats to avoid:

X refined oils such as corn, canola, grape seed oil, rice bran oil, peanut oil, rapeseed oil, soybean oil, cottonseed oil, and sunflower oil.

X also, do away with oils that are purified with the use of hexane solvents, and one that is labeled hydrogenated and partially hydrogenated. These products are linked to cancer producing cells.

It should also be 20% protein. Consuming protein in moderation can help in curbing cravings and will make you feel full for longer hours. Protein is especially beneficial for people who are often working out that helps in sustaining bones and muscles and in burning fats.

This is how you will compute your recommended protein intake per day: your weight multiplied by 0.6 for the minimum grams of protein per day, and then your weight multiplied by 1.0 if you want to get the maximum grams of protein per day.

Take a look at these:

150 pounds x 0.6 = 90 grams (minimum)

150 pounds x 1.0 = 150 grams (maximum)

Some of the best sources of proteins for the ketogenic diet are:

✓ butter

✓ cottage cheese

✓ buttermilk

✓ goat's cheese

✓ feta cheese

✓ cream cheese

√ sour cream

√ yogurt

√ powdered milk

√ curd

√ kefir milk

√ evaporated milk

√ caught wild such as crab, prawns/shrimps, fish, lobsters, squid, scallops, mussels, clams, and oysters.

√ grass-fed such as beef, organ meat, veal, pork, lamb, goat, chicken, turkey, duck, and their eggs.

√ deli meat is allowed in the ketogenic diet provided that they do not contain sugar and starch such as: roasted ham, chicken ham, turkey sausages, corned beef brisket, smoked bacon, salami, and pancetta.

√ nuts and seeds

Protein to avoid:

X filled milk products

X condensed milk, frozen custard, ice cream, frozen yogurt, etc.

X whey protein

X artificially flavored and pre-seasoned food

10% net carbohydrates. Acceptable, quality carbs should come from fresh produce, specifically non-starchy and brightly-colored fruits and veggies.

What is ketosis?

Ketosis is a metabolic state hat the body enters when the ketone levels in the blood reach around 0.5 mmol/l. The by-product of ketosis are ketones. They are a type of acid that accumulate in the blood, which are eliminated in the urine.

Before the word "acid" sends you to a panic mode, let us clarify that the small amount of ketones are harmless. They come as a result of the body's burning and breaking down of fat. They are an indication of the body entering ketosis. However, if ketone levels are too high, it can cause poisoning and will likely lead to a process known as ketoacidosis.

The body does not enter this metabolic state under normal circumstances with your normal diet. It will however, when you restrict your carb consumption. It can also occur when you start fasting for a couple of days. As long as there's sufficiently available carbs from your diet, your body will refuse to enter this metabolic state. In addition, as long as there's remaining stored glycogen in the body or stored form of sugar, the body will not go into ketosis. While sugar is available to provide energy to the cells, the body will refuse to take an alternative fuel supply.

The truth is the body is fine with using glucose as the primary source of fuel. A lot of people never enter the state of ketosis in their lifetime and they still manage to be at an optimum health. Now, you may ask, if you can be at an optimal health without ketosis then what is the purpose of forcing the body to enter ketosis?

What is the purpose of ketosis?

To understand the health purpose of ketosis, a comparison between ketones and sugar will be helpful.

Ketones help the body. And it goes deeper than simply weight loss. It makes the human body work better in the following ways.

-ketones provide a more efficient source of energy.

-they can help resist aging.

-ketones can protect the brain and help prevent neurological disorders.

Ketones possesses unique properties that sugar can't. For one thing, ketones are processed and burned in a more efficient manner than sugar ever could. This means ketones are much better as a provider of a more efficient energy source. They also form less reactive oxygen agents. Moreover, ketones have the ability to elevate mitochondrial production and efficiency. This in turn, helps in enhancing the ketone burning cell's ability of producing energy. It also aids in slowing down the process of aging.

According to research, ketones can also act as a neuroprotective antioxidant. It can support in the reversal and prevention of brain damage. At the same time, it triggers the creation of new brain cells and proliferation of connection between brain cells. The process of ketone burning causes a shift of balance in the brain's neurotransmitters, glutamate and gaba. Excessive neuronal activity can lead to uncontrollable behaviors. This is common among people suffering from neurological disorders such as parkinson's, autism and epilepsy.

By improving the neurotransmitter balance, ketones assist in protecting the brain from excessive neuronal activity which is helpful for preventing neurological disorders. There are studies that also delve into the way ketosis and ketones can be an effective part of treatment for people suffering from alzheimer's and certain types of cancer.

Chapter 2. Pro Tips To Make The Perfect Bread

Whether you're just baking bread for the first time or you just want to bake better goodies, this will give you all kinds of helpful insight to ensure that you make the most of your baking. From important elements to quick fixes and even simple basics, you'll find it all here.

Measurements make a difference

When it comes to baking, measurements are not merely a suggestion. Rather, they are a science. You have to be very careful about measuring out your ingredients. For starters, make sure that you go to a kitchen store or shop online to supply your kitchen with actual measuring tools. Make sure that you have liquid and dry measuring tools in various sizes.

The biggest mistakes that you want to avoid include:

Don't use liquid measures for dry ingredients, and vice versa

Tablespoons and teaspoons are interchangeable for liquid and dry. Cups, however, are not. If you need two cups of water, it needs to be two liquid cups. Don't believe there's a difference? Use a dry cup measure and fill it with water. Then, pour it into your liquid measuring cup. You'll quickly see that the measurement is less than exact.

Don't skip the salt!

Unless you are specifically altering a recipe for sodium content (in which case you should find a low or no sodium version), salt is an ingredient for a reason and you cannot leave it out. Even if it seems like it wouldn't make a difference, it could ruin a recipe.

Get a conversion chart, app, or magnet for the fridge

There are plenty of kitchen conversion guides out there that you can keep on hand. That way, if you need to convert measurements or make substitutions, you know exactly how to do it. You'll find all of your cooking and baking to be more enjoyable when you have conversions and substitutions at hand at all times.

If you're still in the beginner stages, you'll want to stick to the book as best as you can until you get the hang of things. Once you branch out and start to experiment, you can toss these rules out the window (except the liquid/dry measure one). The deliciousness of baking is in the details, and you cannot afford to make simple mistakes when it comes to measurements. There is a reason for the recipe, so if you want to get the best result, follow the directions to the letter.

Quality matters

When you are baking anything, the quality of the ingredients that you use will make a difference. It isn't to say that the store brand flour isn't as good as the name brand because it very well might be. However, you should be careful in choosing higher quality ingredients in order to get better results. If you have the choice, go to a baker's supply or a local bakery outlet to buy the good stuff at better prices. If not, make sure that you get to know your basic ingredients and which ones are best.

The more familiar you get with your own baking abilities and preferences, the more you will be able to decide for yourself where quality matters most. Until then, keep these tips in mind. Also, remember that higher protein content counts with your flour if you're baking bread. More protein means stronger gluten, which makes better bread. Cake flour has a softer texture and lower protein count, which makes it ideal for baking cakes and other desserts.

Recipes all have a reason

A lot of people prefer just to "throw in" the ingredients or measure hastily, which is fine if you're an expert or you're baking something that you've made 100 times before. If, however, you are trying to replicate something out of a recipe book, you need to follow the recipe. Even a single missed ingredient or mismeasurement can turn your bread into something completely different than what you wanted.

It's not like you are going to ruin everything by taking on baking with reckless abandon. If you're new at the bread machine game, though, you should get used to what you're doing before you throw caution to the wind and throw the recipe aside once you remind yourself of the baking temperature.

Even if you concoct your own recipes over time, you'll want to write down at least a rough estimate of what the measurement is. It's hard to share recipes that don't have finite measurements. While you might know exactly how much a "little" salt is, other people can't measure that accurately. Cooking takes skill, but baking is a science, and it should be treated as such.

Stop: check your settings

Again, the process is important. In that, you should also be sure that you check the settings of your bread machine before you start any new baking program. Even if you think you left it on the right setting or programmed the right feature, you need to double check every time. There is nothing worse than waiting an entire hour to realize that you've been using the wrong setting. At that point, your recipe will most likely be ruined.

For beginners, the pre-programmed settings should be perfect, for the most part. There are a lot more options for those who are more experienced with bread machines like the bread machine, and everyone will get there eventually. When in doubt, use the programs and features on the machine, and let it make the hard decisions for you. You'll get great results and if the program isn't exactly right, you'll at least have a starting point to begin making adjustments.

Buttermilk basics

Some people might not even understand exactly what buttermilk is. You don't have to be embarrassed; a lot of people don't know what this weird baking ingredient is for. Buttermilk, traditionally, was what was left after the cream was churned into butter. Most of the buttermilk that you find on the shelves today is cultured or made.

Buttermilk is used because it adds a slight tang to baked goods. It also increases the rise of the bread or pastry by reacting with the baking soda in the recipe. Buttermilk is in a lot of bread and dessert recipes. However, not everyone just happens to keep buttermilk around. If you aren't in the habit of keeping it around, or if you decide to bake something at the last minute, there is a solution. You can take a liquid measuring cup (one cup is fine). In a measuring cup, add a tablespoon of lemon juice in the. Next, add milk up to half cup mark. Allow it to sit for a little bit, and voila, you have homemade buttermilk.

Try something new

Experimenting is good. If you're a novice at baking bread or just starting to learn your bread machine, you might not want to stray too far from the traditional. However, if you are willing to make mistakes for the sake of success, experiment away! As you get more experienced in baking breads with your bread machine, you will be more comfortable in changing things up and seeing what all you can make on your own.

Consistency checks

The big difference with baking bread, compared to other cooking, is that you need to keep an eye on the consistency. While the good old "lightly brown" rule does stand in most cases, the consistency can be very different in a bread machine like the bread machine. Make sure that you capitalize on that "pause" feature and give yourself the chance to check in on your baked goods from time to time to ensure that they turn out their best.

You don't need to interrupt your baking processes too often. Once should be enough. When you're making bread, it's a great idea to pause to remove the paddle, and at the same time, check on the bread and see how it's coming along. Not only does that allow you to ensure that the consistency is right, but it also allows you to get that paddle out before it's baked into the loaf and becomes a chore to remove.

Chapter 3. Ingredients And Tool Used

There are many types of keto bread for you to bake at home. As a result, there are many varying recipes of keto bread for you to pick from. Here are the main keto bread ingredients-

Butter

Butter has saturated fats, compared to carbohydrates and proteins, and a higher concentration of calories. It is a very versatile ingredient regardless of the recipe. It can be used in cooking, spreading, and baking. There are also different types of butter used in the keto diet. They are ghee, grass-fed butter, and clarified butter. Clarified butter is total fat without milk, lactose, or protein. It is good for an individual who is lactose intolerant. Ghee takes a bit longer to prepare compared to clarified butter. Grass-fed butter is the best since it contains higher levels of conjugated linoleic acid compared to commercial butter. Conjugated linoleic acid assists consumers in losing body fat.

Flour

You can use coconut flour, flax meal, ground flaxseed, almond meal, or almond flour when baking your keto bread. Remember, almond meal and almond flour are two different things. The almond meal is prepared from whole almonds, and the skin is removed to prepare the almond flour.

Coconut flour is another alternative to the wheat flour. The coconut flour is produced from coconut pulp after the raw product has been processed for its milk. Rich in fiber, healthy fats, and proteins, coconut flour is good for baking. However, because it has high fiber concentration, it is denser than regular flour. So you have to measure it exactly and work with a given ratio. When working on a given recipe requiring you to substitute wheat flour for coconut flour, the ratio will be 1:4. For a cup of regular wheat flour, you will substitute it with only a quarter cup of coconut flour.

Additionally, using eggs is important when using coconut flour. Eggs are a binding factor for the ingredients giving a good structure. Not using eggs will lead to poor cohesion and cause your meal to crumble. Use an egg for every quarter cup of coconut flour.

Macadamia nuts and flax seeds are two sources of keto flour. Flaxseeds are rich in dietary fiber and omega-3 fats. They are known as flax meal when consumed whole.

Sweeteners

Sweeteners can be used as a substitute for sugar. Remember, not all sweeteners are low-carb. For example, honey, a natural sweetener has more carb content than sugar. The keto sweeteners you can use for baking are monk fruit, erythritol, and stevia. They neither bring digestive complications nor increase your blood sugar levels. Obtained from plants, stevia, and monk fruit sweetener are natural sweeteners. Some people complain that stevia has a rather bitter aftertaste, but monk fruit sweetener has no aftertaste to it. Erythritol is a sugar alcohol produced from the fermentation of corn or birch. It has a cooling effect similar to mint, but you don't have to worry.

Baking powder

Use aluminum-free baking powder. Using aluminum-free baking powder ensures that you don't taste the baking powder when eating the bread.

Chapter 4. Essential Recipes

Basil Cheese Bread

Preparation time: 5 minutes

Cooking time: 15 minutes

Servings: 10

Ingredients

☐ almond flour, two cups

☐ warm water, one cup

☐ salt, half a teaspoon

☐ basil dried, one teaspoon

☐ half cup of mozzarella shredded cheese

☐ quarter tsp. Of active dry yeast

☐ 3 tsp. Of melted unsalted butter

☐ 1 tsp. Of stevia powder

Directions

In a mixing container, combine the almond flour, dried basil, salt, shredded mozzarella cheese, and stevia powder.

Get another container, where you will combine the warm water and the melted unsalted butter.

As per the instructions on the manual of your machine, pour the ingredients in the bread pan, taking care to follow how to mix in the yeast.

Place the bread pan in the machine, and select the sweet bread setting, together with the crust type, if available, then press start once you have closed the lid of the machine.

When the bread is ready, using oven mitts, remove the bread pan from the machine. Use a stainless spatula to extract the bread from the pan and turn the pan upside down on a metallic rack where the bread will cool off before slicing it.

Nutrition:

Calories: 124

Fat: 8g

Carb: 2g

Protein: 11g

American Cheese Beer Bread

Preparation time: 5 minutes

Cooking time: 15 minutes

Servings: 10

Ingredients

☐ 1 ½ cups of fine almond flour

☐ 3 tsp. Of unsalted melted butter

☐ salt, one teaspoon

☐ an egg

☐ swerve sweetener, two teaspoons

☐ keto low-carb beer, one cup

☐ ¾ tsp. Of baking powder

☐ ½ cup of cheddar cheese, shredded

☐ ½ tsp. Of active dry yeast

Directions

Prepare a mixing container, where you will combine the almond flour, swerve sweetener, salt, shredded cheddar cheese, and baking powder.

Prepare another mixing container, where you will combine the unsalted melted butter, egg, and low-carb keto beer.

As per the instructions on the manual of your machine, pour the ingredients in the bread pan, taking care to follow how to mix in the yeast.

Place the bread pan in the machine, and select the basic bread setting, together with the bread size and crust type, if available, then press start once you have closed the lid of the machine.

When the bread is ready, using oven mitts, remove the bread pan from the machine. Use a stainless spatula to extract the bread from the pan and turn the pan upside down on a metallic rack where the bread will cool off before slicing it.

Nutrition:

Calories: 94

Fat: 6g

Carb: 4g

Protein: 1g

Parmesan Cheddar Bread

Preparation time: 5 minutes

Cooking time: 15 minutes

Servings: 10

Ingredients

☐ parmesan cheese grated, one cup

☐ almond flour, one cup

☐ baking powder, half a teaspoon

☐ salt, 3/4 teaspoon

☐ cayenne pepper, a quarter teaspoon

☐ unsweetened almond milk half a cup

☐ sour cream, a third cup full

☐ active dry yeast, one teaspoon

☐ 2 tsp. Of unsalted melted butter

☐ 1 egg

Directions

Get a container for mixing, and combine the almond flour, shredded parmesan cheese, cayenne pepper, baking powder, and salt.

In another mixing container, combine the unsweetened almond milk, sour cream, egg, and unsalted melted butter.

As per the instructions on the manual of your machine, pour the ingredients in the bread pan, taking care to follow how to mix in the yeast.

Place the bread pan in the machine, and select the basic bread setting, together with the bread size and crust type, if available, then press start once you have closed the lid of the machine.

When the bread is ready, using oven mitts, remove the bread pan from the machine. Use a stainless spatula to extract the bread from the pan and turn the pan upside down on a metallic rack where the bread will cool off before slicing it.

Nutrition:

Calories: 134

Fat: 6.8g

Carb: 4.2g

Protein: 12.1g

Pepper Cheddar Bread

Preparation time: 5 minutes

Cooking time: 15 minutes

Servings: 10

Ingredients

☐ ½ cup of coconut flour

☐ 1 cup of almond blanched fine flour

☐ 1 tsp. Of black pepper powder

- ☐ ¾ cup of warm water

- ☐ cheese of cheddar grated, one cup

- ☐ salt, one teaspoon

- ☐ unsalted melted butter, two teaspoons

- ☐ baking powder, one teaspoon

- ☐ active dry yeast, one teaspoon

Directions

Get a container for mixing, and combine the almond flour, coconut flour, shredded cheddar cheese, black pepper powder, baking powder, and salt.

Get another container, where you will combine the warm water and unsalted melted butter.

As per the instructions on the manual of your machine, pour the ingredients in the bread pan, taking care to follow how to mix in the yeast.

Place the bread pan in the machine, and select the basic bread setting, together with the bread size and crust type, if available, then press start once you have closed the lid of the machine.

When the bread is ready, using oven mitts, remove the bread pan from the machine.

Use a stainless spatula to extract the bread from the pan and turn the pan upside down on a metallic rack where the bread will cool off before slicing it.

Nutrition:

Calories: 84

Fat: 4g

Carb: 3g

Protein: 1g

Olive Cheese Bread

Preparation time: 5 minutes

Cooking time: 15 minutes

Servings: 10

Ingredients

- ☐ almond flour, one cup

- ☐ coconut flour, a third cup full

- ☐ olives black halved, a full cup

- ☐ olives green halved, a full cup

- ☐ baking powder, one teaspoon

- ☐ active dry yeast, one teaspoon

- ☐ almond milk, unsweetened, a third cup full

- ☐ shredded mozzarella cheese, two-thirds of a cup

- ☐ ¼ cup of melted unsalted butter

- ☐ ¼ cup of chopped green onions

- ☐ 1/3 cup of mayonnaise

Directions

In a mixing container, combine the almond flour, coconut flour, shredded mozzarella cheese, chopped green onions, chopped black olives, chopped green olives, and baking powder.

Prepare another mixing container, where you will combine the unsweetened almond milk, mayonnaise, and melted unsalted butter.

As per the instructions on the manual of your machine, pour the ingredients in the bread pan, taking care to follow how to mix in the yeast.

Place the bread pan in the machine, and select the basic bread setting, together with the bread size and crust type, if available, then press start once you have closed the lid of the machine.

When the bread is ready, extract it, and place it on a metallic mesh surface to cool completely before cutting and eating it.

Nutrition:

Calories: 134

Fat: 6.8g

Carb: 4.2g

Protein: 12.1g

Feta Oregano Bread

Preparation time: 5 minutes

Cooking time: 15 minutes

Servings: 10

Ingredients

☐ almond flour, one cup

☐ crumbled feta cheese, one cup

☐ half cup of warm water

☐ oregano dried, one teaspoon

- □ baking powder, two-thirds of a teaspoon

- □ extra virgin olive oil, a teaspoon

- □ salt, half a teaspoon

- □ swerve sweetener, one teaspoon

- □ garlic powder, a quarter teaspoon

- □ dried active yeast, one teaspoon

Directions

In a mixing container, combine the almond flour, swerve sweetener, dried oregano, baking powder, ground garlic, and salt.

In another mixing container, combine the extra virgin olive oil and warm water.

As per the instructions on the manual of your machine, pour the ingredients in the bread pan, taking care to follow how to mix in the yeast.

Place the bread pan in the machine, and select the sweet bread setting, together with the bread size and crust type, if available, then press start once you have closed the lid of the machine.

When the bread is ready, using oven mitts, remove the bread pan from the machine. Use a stainless spatula to extract the bread from the pan and turn the pan upside down on a metallic rack where the bread will cool off before slicing it.

Nutrition:

Calories: 114

Fat: 7g

Carb: 8g

Protein: 9g

Goat Cheese Bread

Preparation time: 5 minutes

Cooking time: 15 minutes

Servings: 10

Ingredients

- ☐ 1 cup of almond blanched fine flour

- ☐ ½ cup of soy flour

- ☐ ¼ of salt

- ☐ 2 tsp. Of fresh thyme, crushed

- ☐ ½ cup of coconut milk, melted

- ☐ 1 tsp. Of pepper cayenne

- ☐ eggs, two

- ☐ mustard of dijon, one teaspoon

- ☐ crumbled fresh goat cheese, one cup

- ☐ baking powder, one teaspoon

- ☐ olive oil, extra virgin, a third cup full

- ☐ active dry yeast, one teaspoon

Directions

Get a mixing container and combine the almond flour, soy flour, fresh thyme, cayenne pepper, salt, crumbled fresh goat cheese, and baking powder.

Get another mixing container and combine extra virgin olive oil, eggs, coconut milk, and dijon mustard.

As per the instructions on the manual of your machine, pour the ingredients in the bread pan, taking care to follow how to mix in the yeast.

Place the bread pan in the machine, and select the basic bread setting, together with the bread size and crust type, if available, then press start once you have closed the lid of the machine.

When the bread is ready, using oven mitts, remove the bread pan from the machine. Use a stainless spatula to extract the bread from the pan and turn the pan upside down on a metallic rack where the bread will cool off before slicing it.

Nutrition:

Calories: 134

Fat: 6.8g

Carb: 4.2g

Protein: 12.1g

Mozzarella Herbs Bread

Preparation time: 5 minutes

Cooking time: 15 minutes

Servings: 10

Ingredients

☐ grated cheese mozzarella, one cup

- [ ] grated cheese parmesan, half a cup

- [ ] salt, half a teaspoon

- [ ] baking powder, one teaspoon

- [ ] almond flour, one cup

- [ ] coconut flour, one cup

- [ ] warm water, half a cup

- [ ] stevia, one teaspoon

- [ ] thyme, dried, a quarter teaspoon

- [ ] garlic, ground, one teaspoon

- [ ] basil, dried, one teaspoon

- [ ] olive oil, extra virgin, one teaspoon

- [ ] unsalted melted butter, two teaspoons

- [ ] a third cup of unsweetened almond milk

Directions

In a mixing container, mix the almond flour, baking powder, salt, parmesan cheese, mozzarella cheese, coconut flour, dried basil, dried thyme, garlic powder, and stevia powder.

Get another mixing container and mix warm water, unsweetened almond milk, melted unsalted butter, and extra virgin olive oil.

As per the instructions on the manual of your machine, pour the ingredients in the bread pan, taking care to follow how to mix in the yeast.

Place the bread pan in the machine, and select the basic bread setting, together with the bread size and crust type, if available, then press start once you have closed the lid of the machine.

When the bread is ready, using oven mitts, remove the bread pan from the machine. Use a stainless spatula to extract the bread from the pan and turn the pan upside down on a metallic rack where the bread will cool off before slicing it.

Nutrition:

Calories: 49

Fat: 2g

Carb: 2g

Protein: 1g

Blue Cheese Onion Bread

Preparation time: 5 minutes

Cooking time: 15 minutes

Servings: 10

Ingredients

☐ half a cup of blue cheese, crumbled

☐ 1 tsp. Of unsalted melted butter

☐ 2 tsp. Of fresh rosemary, chopped

☐ 1 ½ cup of almond fine flour

☐ olive oil extra virgin, two teaspoons

☐ baking powder, one teaspoon

☐ warm water, half a cup

☐ a yellow onion sliced and sautéed in butter until golden brown

☐ 2 garlic cloves, crushed

☐ yeast, one teaspoon

☐ swerve sweetener, one teaspoon

☐ salt, one teaspoon

Directions

Prepare a mixing container, where you will combine the almond flour, swerve sweetener, baking powder, freshly chopped rosemary, crumbled blue cheese, sautéed sliced onion, salt, and crushed garlic.

Get another container, where you will combine the warm water, melted butter, and extra virgin olive oil.

As per the instructions on the manual of your machine, pour the ingredients in the bread pan, taking care to follow how to mix in the yeast.

Place the bread pan in the machine, and select the basic bread setting, together with the bread size and crust type, if available, then press start once you have closed the lid of the machine.

When the bread is ready, using oven mitts, remove the bread pan from the machine. Use a stainless spatula to extract the bread from the pan, and turn the pan upside down on a metallic rack where the bread will cool off before slicing it.

Nutrition:

Calories: 100

Fat: 6g Carb: 3g

Protein: 11g

Low-Carb Bagel

Preparation time: 15 minutes

Cooking time: 25 minutes

Servings: 12

Ingredients

☐ 1 cup protein powder, unflavored

☐ 1/3 cup coconut flour

☐ 1 tsp. Baking powder

☐ ½ tsp. Sea salt

☐ ¼ cup ground flaxseed

☐ 1/3 cup sour cream

☐ 12 eggs

Seasoning topping:

☐ 1 tsp. Dried parsley

☐ 1 tsp. Dried oregano

☐ 1 tsp. Dried minced onion

☐ ½ tsp. Garlic powder

☐ ½ tsp. Dried basil

☐ ½ tsp. Sea salt

Directions

Preheat the oven to 350f.

In a mixer, blend sour cream and eggs until well combined.

Whisk together the flaxseed, salt, baking powder, protein powder, and coconut flour in a bowl.

Gently mix the dry ingredients into the wet ingredients until well blended.

Whisk the topping seasoning together in a small bowl. Set aside.

Grease 2 donut pans that can contain 6 donuts each.

Sprinkle pan with about 1 tsp. Topping seasoning and evenly pour batter into each.

Sprinkle the top of each bagel evenly with the rest of the seasoning mixture.

Bake in the oven for 25 minutes, or until golden brown.

Cool and serve.

Nutrition:

Calories: 134

Fat: 6.8g

Carb: 4.2g

Protein: 12.1g

Cheddar Sausage Biscuits

Preparation time: 15 minutes

Cooking time: 25 minutes

Servings: 8

Ingredients

☐ 6 oz. Cooked sausage, grease drained, thinly sliced

☐ ¼ cup water

☐ ¼ cup heavy cream

☐ 1 cup shredded sharp white cheddar cheese

☐ 1 ½ cups almond flour

☐ ½ tsp. Italian seasoning

☐ ½ tsp. Sea salt

☐ 1 tbsp. Chopped fresh chives

☐ 2 minced large garlic cloves

☐ 1 large egg

☐ 4 oz. Softened cream cheese

Directions

Preheat the oven to 350f.

Using a hand mixer on low speed, whip the eggs and cream cheese in a bowl.

Add the garlic, chives, sea salt, italian seasoning, then mix into the egg cheese mixture.

Add the water, almond flour, heavy cream, and cheddar cheese. Mix well.

Slowly mix in the sausage into the mixture using a spatula.

Lightly grease muffin pan.

Drop a heap mold of dough into 8 wells on the muffin top pan.

Bake in the oven for 25 minutes.

Cool and serve.

Nutrition:

Calories: 321 Fat: 28g Carb: 3.5g Protein: 13g

Low-Carb Pretzels

Preparation time: 15 minutes

Cooking time: 15 minutes

Servings: 12

Ingredients

☐ 1 tbsp. Pretzel salt

☐ 2 tbsp. Butter, melted

☐ 2 tbsp. Warm water

☐ 2 tsp. Dried yeast

☐ 2 eggs

☐ 2 tsp. Xanthan gum

- 1 ½ cups almond flour

- 4 tbsp. Cream cheese

- 3 cups of shredded mozzarella cheese

Directions

Preheat the oven to 390f.

Melt the mozzarella cheese and cream cheese in the microwave.

Combine warm water with yeast and let sit for 2 minutes and activate.

Mix the almond meal and xanthan gum with a hand mixer.

Add yeast mixture, 1 tbsp. Melted butter, and eggs and mix well.

Add in the melted cheese and knead the dough, about 5 to 10 minutes or until well combined.

Divide into 12 balls while the dough is still warm, then roll into a long, thin log and then twist to form a pretzel shape.

Transfer onto a lined cookie sheet, leaving small space between them.

Brush the remaining butter on top the pretzels and sprinkle with the salt.

Bake for 12 to 15 minutes in the oven or until golden brown.

Nutrition:

Calories: 217

Fat: 18g

Carb: 3g

Protein: 11g

Shortbread Vanilla Cookies

Preparation time: 15 minutes

Cooking time: 20 minutes

Servings: 16

Ingredients

☐ 1 egg

☐ ½ cup unsalted butter, softened

☐ 1 tsp. Vanilla extract

☐ 1 pinch salt

☐ 1/3 cup erythritol

☐ 2 cups almond flour

Directions

Preheat the oven to 300f.

Mix together the almond flour, erythritol, salt, and vanilla extract in a bowl.

Pour in butter and mix with the almond flour mix unit well combined. Add egg and mix well.

Roll one tbsp. Mixture into a ball. Place them onto a lined cookie sheet with gaps in between. Press.

Place in the oven and bake for 12 to 25 minutes, or until the edges are browned.

Cool and serve.

Nutrition:

Calories: 126 Fat: 12g Carb: 2g Protein: 3g

Low-Carb Taco Shells

Preparation time: 10 minutes

Cooking time: 15 minutes

Servings: 4

Ingredients

☐ ½ tsp. Ground cumin

☐ 8 ounces shredded cheese

Directions

Preheat the oven to 400f.

Mix together the cumin and cheese.

Line a baking sheet with parchment paper.

Drop 6 to 8 heaps of the cheese on the prepared sheet with. Keep enough space between them.

Bake until cheese is bubbling with golden brown patches, about 10 to 15 minutes. Be careful not to burn the cheese.

Allow to cool for half a minute.

Place a rack on the sink and gently arrange cheese tortillas over the rack.

Before cheese cools down completely, let each round's edges drop down between the rack's bars to from taco shell shape.

Nutrition:

Calories: 202

Fat: 16g Carb: 1g Protein: 13g

Keto Buns

Preparation time: 5 minutes

Cooking time: 26 minutes

Servings: 6

Ingredients

- ☐ 1 tsp. Onion flakes

- ☐ 1 tbsp. Black sesame seeds

- ☐ 1 tbsp. White sesame seeds

- ☐ 1 tsp. Rosemary

- ☐ 3.5 oz. Almond flour

- ☐ ½ tsp. Himalayan salt

- ☐ 4 eggs

- ☐ 4 tbsp. Unsalted butter

Directions

Preheat the oven to 430f. Add the eggs and melted butter inside a stick blender beaker. Add the remaining ingredients and place the stick blender into the beaker. Pulse until batter is fully mixed. Take 6 silicone jumbo muffin molds and evenly pour the batter. If desired, sprinkle top of each bun with extra sesame seeds.

Bake in the oven at 430f for 26 minutes.

Cool, slice, and serve.

Nutrition: Calories: 230 Fat: 20.82g Carb: 3.99g Protein: 8.45g

Goat Cheese Crackers

Preparation time: 5 minutes

Cooking time: 20 minutes

Servings: 12

Ingredients

- ☐ 6 oz. Goat cheese

- ☐ ½ cup coconut flour

- ☐ 4 tbsp. Butter

- ☐ 2 tbsp. Fresh rosemary

- ☐ 1 tsp. Baking powder

Directions

In a food processor, combine all ingredients and mix until smooth.

Roll out the dough with a rolling pin to about ¼ to ½ inch thick and cut out the crackers with a knife or cookie cutter.

Line a baking sheet with parchment paper and place the crackers on it.

Bake at 380f for 15 to 20 minutes.

Nutrition:

Calories: 99

Fat: 8g

Carb: 2g Protein: 4g

Chocolate Chip Cookies

Preparation time: 10 minutes

Cooking time: 15 minutes

Servings: 15

Ingredients

- ☐ 1 cup chocolate flour

- ☐ ½ cup butter, softened

- ☐ 1 cup unsweetened coconut flakes

- ☐ 4 eggs

- ☐ 2 2/3 oz. Dark chocolate chips

- ☐ ½ tsp. Vanilla extract

- ☐ ½ cup erythritol

Directions

Mix the erythritol, butter, vanilla, eggs, and salt together.

Add the chocolate chips, coconut flakes, and coconut flour. Mix well.

Line a baking sheet with parchment paper and spoon the cookies onto it.

Bake at 375f for 15 to 20 minutes.

Nutrition:

Calories: 195

Fat: 16g Carb: 5g Protein: 4g

Buns With Cottage Cheese

Preparation time: 10 minutes

Cooking time: 15 minutes

Servings: 8

Ingredients

☐ 2 eggs

☐ 3 oz. Almond flour

☐ 1 oz. Erythritol

☐ 1/8 tsp. Stevia

☐ cinnamon and vanilla extract to taste

Filling:

☐ 5 ½ oz. Cottage cheese

☐ 1 egg

☐ cinnamon and vanilla extract to taste

Directions

Prepare the filling by mixing its ingredients in a bowl.

Combine eggs with almond flour, blend until smooth. Add erythritol, stevia, and flavors to taste.

Spoon 1 tbsp. Dough into silicone cups. Spoon about 1 tsp. Filling on top, and bake at 365f for 15 minutes.

Nutrition: Calories: 77 Fat: 5.2g Carb: 6.7g Protein: 5.8g

Sandwich Buns

Preparation time: 10 minutes

Cooking time: 25 minutes

Servings: 8

Ingredients

☐ 4 eggs

☐ 2 ½ oz. Almond flour

☐ 1 tbsp. Coconut flour

☐ 1 oz. Psyllium

☐ 1 ½ cups eggplant, finely grated, juices drained

☐ 3 tbsp. Sesame seeds

☐ 1 ½ tsp. Baking powder

☐ salt to taste

Directions

Whisk eggs until foamy, and then add grated eggplant.

In a separate bowl, mix all dry ingredients.

Add them to the egg mixture. Mix well.

Line a baking sheet with parchment paper and shape the buns with your hands.

Bake at 374f for 20 to 25 minutes.

Nutrition: Calories: 99 Fat: 6g Carb: 10g Protein: 5.3g

Chapter 5. Ketogenic Gluten Free Bread Recipes

Monkey Bread

Preparation time: 25 minutes

Cooking time: 40 minutes

Servings: 12

Ingredients:

3 large eggs, lightly beaten

½ cup oil

½ cup plus 1 tbsp water

1 cup buttermilk or sour milk

2 cups brown rice flour

½ cup potato starch

½ cup tapioca flour

3½ tsp xanthan gum

½ cup sugar

1½ tsp salt

1 package dry yeast

Sweet dust coating

½ cup rice flour

¼ cup sugar

3 tbsp cinnamon

¼ tsp salt

Directions:

Preheat oven to 400°f.

Grease a bundt pan or an 8-inch cake pan, using a spray of oil or a paper napkin saturated with oil.

Combine wet ingredients in a large bowl or baking pan of a bread maker.

Blend dry ingredients together, including the yeast, in a separate bowl.

Add well-blended dry ingredients to combined wet ingredients.

Select normal/white cycle for bread machine.

Mix all ingredients in the bread machine—use a rubber spatula to scrape the inside edges of the bread machine to incorporate all the mixture. Alternatively, mix all ingredients by hand; let rise till doubled in size.

Remove bread pan after first bake cycle.

Combine sweet dust coating ingredients.

Roll fistfuls of risen dough lightly in sweet coating.

Put the rolls in the cake pan, stuffing all coated balls side by side. (you can knead the remains of the flour, sugar, and cinnamon with softened butter and then sprinkle over tops of the monkey rolls.)

Bake at 400°f for 40 minutes, until a knife comes out clean.

Nutrition: Carbohydrates: 49.6 g Fat:6.8 g Protein:4.8 g Calories:279

Yeast Bread With Molasses

Preparation time: 25 minutes

Cooking time: 40 minutes

Servings: 16 slices

Ingredients:

1 cup brown rice flour

1 cup white rice flour

½ cup tapioca flour

½ cup potato starch flour

½ cup kasha, ground slightly in coffee grinder

2½ tsp xanthan gum

1½ tsp table salt

3 eggs, lightly beaten

1½ cups water

1 tsp vinegar or 1½ tsp dough enhancer (lemon)

3 tbsp olive oil or butter

1 tbsp molasses

3 tbsp sugar

1 tbsp dry yeast

Directions:

Blend together the flours, kasha, xanthan gum, and salt.

Combine the eggs, water, vinegar or dough enhancer, oil, and molasses.

Stir together the sugar and yeast.

Place the ingredients in the baking pan.

Bake in oven at 350°f for 40 minutes until brown.

Nutrition: Carbohydrates: 32.1 g Fat:4.1 g Protein:3.9 g Calories:181

Brown And White Rice Bread

Preparation time: 25 minutes

Cooking time: 1 hour

Servings: 15 slices

Ingredients:

2½ cups white rice flour

1 cup brown rice flour

2½ tsp xanthan gum

3 tbsp sugar

1½ tsp salt

½ cup dry milk

2 packages active dry yeast

½ cup golden raisins

3 eggs, lightly beaten

1 tsp cider vinegar

3 tbsp canola oil

1½ cups water

Directions:

Preheat oven to 325°f. Grease bottom of 9 x 5 x 3-inch loaf pan.

Mix the dry and wet ingredients in separate bowls.

Add wet ingredients to dry and stir just until it reaches the consistency of cake batter.

Put in loaf pan.

Proof for 15 minutes in a warm oven. Let it rise.

Bake in oven at 325°f for 1 hour.

Nutrition:

Carbohydrates: 36.5 g

Fat:0 g

Protein:5.1 g

Calories:215

Chickpea Yeast Bread

Preparation time: 15 minutes

Cooking time: 1 hour

Servings: 15 slices

Ingredients:

3 large eggs, lightly beaten

1 tsp cider vinegar

3 tbsp olive oil

1½ cups water

1 tsp pure maple syrup

1 cup chickpea flour

1 cup brown rice flour

1 cup tapioca flour

½ cup cornstarch

3 tsp xanthan gum

3 tbsp brown sugar

2 tsp sea salt

½ cup dry milk

1 package dry yeast

Directions:

Grease bottom of 9 x 5 x 3-inch loaf pan.

Mix the dry and wet ingredients in separate bowls.

Add wet ingredients to dry and stir just until cake-batter consistency.

Put in loaf pan.

Proof for 45 minutes or longer in a barely warm oven; let rise slightly.

Remove from oven and let stand for 15 minutes.

Preheat oven to 325°f.

Bake for 1 hour. If it browns too quickly, cover with a piece of aluminum foil, shiny-side up.

Nutrition: Carbohydrates: 30.8 g Fat:5.6 g Protein:4.9 g Calories:194

Farmhouse Sour Milk Yeast Bread

Preparation time: 25 minutes

Cooking time: 1 hour

Servings: 15 slices

Ingredients:

3 large eggs, lightly beaten

½ cup oil

½ cup plus 1 tbsp water

1 cup buttermilk

1 cup garbanzo and/or fava bean flour

1 cup millet flour

½ cup potato starch

½ cup tapioca flour

3½ tsp xanthan gum

½ cup sugar

1½ tsp salt

2 tsp powdered eggs

1 package dry yeast

Directions:

Grease 9 x 5 x 3-inch loaf pan.

Mix the wet ingredients together.

Mix the dry ingredients together in a separate bowl.

Add blended dry ingredient to blended wet ingredients, bit by bit, by hand. Stir just until combined.

Put in loaf pan.

Proof at room temperature all day or in a warm oven for 45 minutes until it rises.

Preheat oven to 325°f.

Bake at for 1 hour.

Nutrition:

Carbohydrates: 33.4 g

Fat:7.7 g Protein:6.8 g Calories:231

Cranberry Yeast Bread

Preparation time: 15 minutes

Cooking time: 10 minutes

Servings: 16 slices

Ingredients:

3 tbsp sugar

1 cup white rice flour

2 cups millet, sorghum, or amaranth flour

¼ cup soy flour

1 tbsp xanthan gum

1½ tsp salt

½ cup dry milk

1 package dry yeast

1 cup dried or fresh cranberries or currants

3 large eggs, lightly beaten

1 tsp cider vinegar

3 tbsp oil

1½ cups water

4 tbsp honey

Directions:

Preheat oven to 350°f.

Grease 9 x 5 x 3- inch loaf pan.

Mix dry ingredients together.

Mix wet ingredients together.

Add dry ingredients to the wet ingredients bit by bit. Stir by hand.

Place in prepared loaf pan.

Let rise all day or overnight.

Cut diagonal slashes into the top of the loaf.

Bake at 350°f for 45 minutes. Turn on side to rest after baking.

Nutrition: Carbohydrates: 30.1 g Fat:5.9 g Protein:5.8 g Calories:197

Pumpkin Yeast Bread

Preparation time: 25 minutes

Cooking time: 45 minutes

Servings: 16 slices

Ingredients:

½ cup warm water

2 cups fresh pumpkin, cooked and mashed

2 cups apple juice, heated to hot in microwave

½ cup canola oil

½ tsp sugar

2 packages dry powdered yeast

2 cups quinoa flour

1 cup soy flour

½ cup tapioca flour

½ cup garbanzo and/or fava bean flour

3 tsp xanthan gum

2 tbsp brown sugar

1 tsp cumin

2 tsp salt

½ cup golden raisins

Directions:

Preheat oven to 350°f.

Grease 9 x 5 x 3- inch loaf pan.

Add warm water and sugar to yeast in a glass measuring cup, cover, and let it proof.

Combine dry ingredients.

Combine pumpkin, apple juice, oil, and raisins.

Stir dry ingredients into pumpkin mixture until the dough looks like cake batter.

Place dough in prepared loaf pan.   Proof with a cloth over dough at room temperature until dough comes to the top of the pan. Bake 45 minutes.

Nutrition: Carbohydrates: 31.7 g Fat:9.2 g Protein:4.9 g Calories:228

Indian Ricegrass Yeast Bread

Preparation time: 25 minutes

Cooking time: 50 minutes

Servings: 15 slices

Ingredients:

2 tsp dry yeast

1 cup gf montina (indian rice grass) flour

1 cup brown rice flour

½ cup soy flour

½ cup cornmeal or quinoa flour

1½ tsp sea salt

½ cup sunflower seeds, ground

2½ cups water

½ cup canola oil

1½ tbsp honey

Topping:

2 tbsp butter, melted

2 tbsp pure sesame seeds

Directions:

Dissolve yeast in warm water. Let rise.

Stir oil and honey into risen yeast mixture.

Mix flours, salt, and ground sunflower seeds together.

Add three-quarters of the flour mixture to the oil-honey-yeast mixture; then add more gradually until dough is smooth and elastic.

Let rise in bowl for 1 hour until doubled in height. Punch down. Add a bit more white rice flour, knead and form into loaves.

Let rise again in a warm place, 45 minutes, with a damp cloth over it.

Preheat oven to 400°f.

Top loaves with melted butter and sesame seeds. Bake for 50 minutes.

Nutrition: Carbohydrates: 23.2 g Fat:8.6 g Protein:5 g Calories:191

Buckwheat Yeast Bread

Preparation time: 20 minutes

Cooking time: 45 minutes

Servings: 12 slices

Ingredients:

½ cup (60 ml) water, very warm

3 eggs, beaten

1½ cups milk

2 tbsp unsulfured molasses

3 tbsp butter, melted

½ cup buckwheat flour

½ cup tapioca flour

1 package (0.25oz) dry yeast

Pinch sugar

1½ cups brown rice flour

½ cup potato starch

1 tsp sea salt

1 tbsp xanthan gum

1 tsp cardamom

Directions:

Grease 9 x 5 x 3-inch loaf pan.

Mix yeast, sugar, and water in a glass measuring cup. Cover with a paper towel and let the yeast rise to the top of the cup.

Stir yeast mixture into beaten eggs.

Add milk, molasses, and melted butter.

Add dry ingredients into wet, a third at a time, stirring with a large wooden spoon or your hands until the batter becomes rich and cake-like.

Cover with a damp cloth and let rise all day or overnight at room temperature. It will taste better the longer it proofs.

Preheat oven to 400°f. Score top of the risen loaf with diagonal cuts. Bake the loaf for about 30-45 minutes.

Nutrition: Carbohydrates: 20.8 g Fat:5.3 g Protein:3.5 g Calories:145

Mock Black Russian Yeast Bread

Preparation time: 20 minutes

Cooking time: 4 hours

Servings: 16 slices

Ingredients:

3 eggs

1 tsp cider vinegar

3 tbsp olive oil

2 tbsp molasses

1½ cups water

2 cups brown rice flour

½ cup potato starch

½ cup tapioca flour

½ cup rice bran

1 tbsp xanthan gum

3 tsp dark brown sugar

1½ tsp salt

½ cup dry milk

1 tbsp instant coffee

4 ½ tsp pure cocoa

2 tbsp caraway seeds

1 package dry yeast

Directions:

Grease 9 x 5 x 3-inch loaf pan.

Mix wet ingredients together.

Whisk dry ingredients together.

Add the mixed dry ingredients to the mixed wet ingredients gradually, by hand. Stir well.

Put into prepared loaf pan.

Proof all day or overnight at room temperature.

Bake at 325°f for 3-4 hours. Test with a toothpick in the center.

Nutrition:

Carbohydrates: 31.3 g

Fat:5.8 g

Protein:4.5 g

Calories:196

Millet Bread

Preparation time: 15 minutes

Cooking time: 30 minutes

Servings: 12 slices

Ingredients:

1 cup plain gf yogurt or buttermilk

½ cup butter

½ cup warm water

1 tbsp honey

2 eggs, beaten

1 package dry yeast

2 cups millet flour

½ cup soy flour

2½ tsp xanthan gum

½ tsp salt

¾ cup millet seeds, crushed or ground, divided

Directions:

Grease 9 x 5 x 3-inch loaf pan with canola oil.

Combine yogurt and butter in a saucepan over low heat, stirring, just until butter is melted.

Dissolve the yeast into the warm water.

Stir in honey and beaten eggs.

Mix yogurt and butter into the yeast mixture.

Add flours, xanthan gum, salt, and ½ cup millet seeds into the wet ingredients slowly, bit by bit, by hand.

Spoon dough into an oiled 9 x 5 x 3-inch bread pan.

Cover and let rise all day at room temperature.

Cut 2 diagonal slashes into top of loaf; sprinkle with remaining ¼ cup millet seeds.

Bake in preheated 375° f oven for 30 minutes

Nutrition:

Carbohydrates: 31.2 g

Fat:6.1 g

Protein:8 g

Calories:212

Chapter 6. Breakfast

Keto Breakfast Bread

Preparation time: 15 minutes

Cooking time: 40 minutes

Servings: 16 slices

Ingredients:

½ tsp. Xanthan gum

½ tsp. Salt

2 tbsp. Coconut oil

½ cup butter, melted

1 tsp. Baking powder - 2 cups of almond flour - 7 eggs

Directions:

1. preheat the oven to 355f.

2. beat eggs in a bowl on high for 2 minutes.

3. add coconut oil and butter to the eggs and continue to beat.

4. line a loaf pan with baking paper and pour the beaten eggs.

5. pour in the rest of the ingredients and mix until it becomes thick.

6. bake until a toothpick comes out dry, about 40 to 45 minutes.

Nutrition: Calories: 234 Fat: 23g Carb: 1g Protein: 7g

Chia Seed Bread

Preparation time: 10 minutes

Cooking time: 40 minutes

Servings: 16 slices

Ingredients

½ tsp. Xanthan gum

½ cup butter

2 tbsp. Coconut oil

1 tbsp. Baking powder

3 tbsp. Sesame seeds

2 tbsp. Chia seeds

½ tsp. Salt

¼ cup sunflower seeds

2 cups almond flour

7 eggs

Directions:

1. preheat the oven to 350f.

2. beat eggs in a bowl on high for 1 to 2 minutes.

3. beat in the xanthan gum and combine coconut oil and melted butter into eggs, beating continuously.

4. set aside the sesame seeds, but add the rest of the ingredients.

5. line a loaf pan with baking paper and place the mixture in it. Top the mixture with sesame seeds.

6. bake in the oven until a toothpick inserted comes out clean, about 35 to 40 minutes.

Nutrition:

Calories: 405

Fat: 37g

Carb: 4g

Protein: 14g

Keto Flax Bread

Preparation time: 10 minutes

Cooking time: 18 to 20 minutes

Servings: 8

Directions:

¾ cup of water

200 g ground flax seeds

½ cup psyllium husk powder

1 tbsp. Baking powder

7 large egg whites

3 tbsp. Butter

2 tsp. Salt

¼ cup granulated stevia

1 large whole egg

1 ½ cups whey protein isolate

Ingredients:

1. preheat the oven to 350f.

2. combine together whey protein isolate, psyllium husk, baking powder, sweetener, and salt.

3. in another bowl, mix together the water, butter, egg, and egg whites.

4. slowly add psyllium husk mixture to egg mixture and mix well.

5. lightly grease a bread pan with butter and pour in the batter.

6. bake in the oven until the bread is set, about 18 to 20 minutes.

Nutrition:

Calories: 265.5

Fat: 15.68g

Carb: 1.88g

Protein:24.34 g

Special Keto Bread

Preparation time: 15 minutes

Cooking time: 40 minutes

Servings: 14

Ingredients:

2 tsp. Baking powder

½ cup water

1 tbsp. Poppy seeds

2 cups fine ground almond meal

5 large eggs

½ cup olive oil

½ tsp. Fine himalayan salt

Directions:

Preheat the oven to 400f.

In a bowl, combine salt, almond meal, and baking powder.

Drip in oil while mixing, until it forms a crumbly dough.

Make a little round hole in the middle of the dough and pour eggs into the middle of the dough.

Pour water and whisk eggs together with the mixer in the small circle until it is frothy.

Start making larger circles to combine the almond meal mixture with the dough until you have a smooth and thick batter.

Line your loaf pan with parchment paper.

Pour batter into the prepared loaf pan and sprinkle poppy seeds on top.

Bake in the oven for 40 minutes in the center rack until firm and golden brown.

Cool in the oven for 30 minutes.

Slice and serve.

Nutrition:

Calories: 227

Fat: 21g

Carb: 4g Protein: 7g

Keto Easy Bread

Preparation time: 15 minutes

Cooking time: 45 minutes

Servings: 10

Ingredients:

¼ tsp. Cream of tartar

1 ½ tsp. Baking powder (double acting)

4 large eggs

1 ½ cups vanilla whey protein

¼ cup olive oil

¼ cup coconut milk, unsweetened

½ tsp. Salt

¼ cup unsalted butter, softened

12 oz. Cream cheese, softened

½ tsp. Xanthan gum

½ tsp. Baking soda

Directions:

Preheat oven to 325f.

Layer aluminum foil over the loaf pan and spray with olive oil.

Beat the butter with cream cheese in a bowl until mixed well.

Add oil and coconut milk and blend until mixed. Add eggs, one by one until fully mixed. Set aside.

In a bowl, whisk whey protein, ½ tsp. Xanthan gum, baking soda, cream of tartar, salt, and baking powder.

Add mixture to egg/cheese mixture and slowly mix until fully combined. Don't over blend.

Place in the oven and bake for 40 to 45 minutes, or until golden brown.

Cool, slice, and serve.

Nutrition:

Calories: 294.2

Fat: 24g

Carb: 1.8g

Protein: 17g

Almond Flour Apple Bread Rolls

Preparation time: 10 minutes

Cooking time: 30 minutes

Servings: 6

Ingredients:

1 cup boiling water or as needed

2 cups almond flour

½ cup ground flaxseed

4 tbsp. Psyllium husk powder

1 tbsp. Baking powder

2 tbsp. Olive oil

2 eggs

1 tbsp. Apple cider vinegar

½ tsp. Salt

Directions:

Preheat the oven to 350f.

In a bowl, mix together the almond flour, baking powder, psyllium husk powder, flax-seed flour, and salt.

Add the olive oil and eggs and blend until mixture resembles breadcrumbs, then mix in the apple cider vinegar.

Slowly add boiling water and mix into the mixture. Let stand for half an hour to firm up.

Line parchment paper over the baking tray.

Using your hands, make a ball of the dough.

Transfer dough balls on a baking tray and bake for 30 minutes, or until firm and golden.

Nutrition:

Calories: 301

Fat: 24.1g

Carb: 5g

Protein: 11g

Low Carb Bread

Preparation time: 10 minutes

Cooking time: 21 minutes

Servings: 12

Ingredients:

2 cups mozzarella cheese, grated

8 oz. Cream cheese

Herbs and spices to taste

1 tbsp. Baking powder

1 cup crushed pork rinds

¼ cup parmesan cheese, grated

3 large eggs

Directions:

Preheat oven to 375f.

Line parchment paper over the baking pan.

In a bowl, place cream cheese and mozzarella and microwave for 1 minute on high power. Stir and microwave for 1 minute more. Then stir again.

Stir in egg, parmesan, pork rinds, herbs, spices and baking powder until mixed.

Spread mixture on the baking pan and bake until top is lightly brown, about 15 to 20 minutes.

Cool, slice, and serve.

Nutrition: Calories: 166 Fat: 13g Carb: 1g Protein: 9g

Splendid Low-Carb Bread

Preparation time: 15 minutes

Cooking time: 60 to 70 minutes

Servings: 12

Ingredients:

½ tsp. Herbs, such as basil, rosemary, or oregano

½ tsp. Garlic or onion powder

1 tbsp. Baking powder

5 tbsp. Psyllium husk powder

½ cup almond flour

½ cup coconut flour

¼ tsp. Salt

1 ½ cup egg whites

3 tbsp. Oil or melted butter

2 tbsp. Apple cider vinegar

1/3 to ¾ cup hot water

Directions:

Grease a loaf pan and preheat the oven to 350f.

In a bowl, whisk the salt, psyllium husk powder, onion or garlic powder, coconut flour, almond flour, and baking powder.

Stir in egg whites, oil, and apple cider vinegar. Bit by bit add the hot water, stirring until dough increase in size. Do not add too much water.

Mold the dough into a rectangle and transfer to grease loaf pan.

Bake in the oven for 60 to 70 minutes, or until crust feels firm and brown on top.

Cool and serve.

Nutrition:

Calories: 97

Fat: 5.7g

Carb: 7.5g

Protein: 4.1g

Bread De Soul

Preparation time: 10 minutes

Cooking time: 45 minutes

Servings: 16

Ingredients:

¼ tsp. Cream of tartar

2 ½ tsp. Baking powder

1 tsp. Xanthan gum

1/3 tsp. Baking soda

½ tsp. Salt

1 2/3 cup unflavored whey protein

¼ cup olive oil

¼ cup heavy whipping cream or half and half

2 drops of sweet leaf stevia

4 eggs

¼ cup butter

12 oz. Softened cream cheese

Directions:

Preheat the oven to 325f.

In a bowl, microwave cream cheese and butter for 1 minute.

Remove and blend well with a hand mixer.

Add olive oil, eggs, heavy cream, and few drops of sweetener and blend well.

Blend together the dry ingredients in a separate bowl.

Combine the dry ingredients with the wet ingredients and mix with a spoon. Don't use a hand blender to avoid whipping it too much.

Grease a bread pan and pour the mixture into the pan.

Bake in the oven until golden brown, about 45 minutes.

Cool and serve.

Nutrition: Calories: 200 Fat: 15.2g Carb: 1.8g Protein: 10g

Sandwich Flatbread

Preparation time: 15 minutes

Cooking time: 20 minutes

Servings: 10

Ingredients:

¼ cup water

¼ cup oil

4 eggs

½ tsp. Salt

1/3 cup unflavored whey protein powder

½ tsp. Garlic powder

2 tsp. Baking powder

6 tbsp. Coconut flour

3 ¼ cups almond flour

Directions:

Preheat the oven to 325f.

Combine the dry ingredients in a large bowl and mix with a hand whisk.

Whisk in eggs, oil, and water until combined well.

Place on a piece of large parchment paper and flatten into a rough rectangle. Place another parchment paper on top.

Roll into a large ½ inch to ¾ inch thick rough rectangle. Transfer to the baking sheet and discard the parchment paper on top.

Bake until it is firm to the touch, about 20 minutes.

Cool and cut into 10 portions.

Carefully cut each part into two halves through the bready center. Stuff with your sandwich fillings.

Serve.

Nutrition:

Calories: 316

Fat: 6.8g

Carb: 11g

Protein: 25.9g

Keto Sandwich Bread

Preparation time: 5 minutes

Cooking time: 1 hour

Servings: 12

Ingredients:

1 tsp. Apple cider vinegar

¾ cup water

¼ cup avocado oil

5 eggs

½ tsp. Salt

1 tsp. Baking soda

½ cup coconut flour

2 cups plus 2 tbsp. Almond flour

Directions:

Preheat the oven to 350f and grease a loaf pan.

In a bowl, whisk almond flour, coconut flour, and salt.

In another bowl, separate the egg whites from egg yolks. Set egg whites aside.

In a blender, blend the oil, egg yolks, water, vinegar, and baking soda for 5 minutes on medium speed until combined.

Let the mixture sit for 1 minute then add in the reserved egg whites and mix until frothy, about 10 to 15 seconds.

Add the dry ingredients and process on high for 5 to 10 seconds before batter becomes too thick for the blender. Blend until the batter is smooth.

Transfer batter into the greased loaf pan and smoothen the top.

Bake in the oven until a skewer inserted comes out clean, about 50 to 70 minutes.

Cool, slice, and serve.

Nutrition: Calories: 200g Fat: 7g Carb: 7g Protein: 16g

Coconut Flour Almond Bread

Preparation time: 10 minutes

Cooking time: 30 minutes

Servings: 4

Ingredients:

1 tbsp. Butter, melted

1 tbsp. Coconut oil, melted

6 eggs

1 tsp. Baking soda

2 tbsp. Ground flaxseed

1 ½ tbsp. Psyllium husk powder

5 tbsp. Coconut flour

1 ½ cup almond flour

Directions:

Preheat the oven to 400f.

Mix the eggs in a bowl for a few minutes.

Add in the butter and coconut oil and mix once more for 1 minute.

Add the almond flour, coconut flour, baking soda, psyllium husk, and ground flaxseed to the mixture. Let sit for 15 minutes.

Lightly grease the loaf pan with coconut oil. Pour the mixture in the pan.

Place in the oven and bake until a toothpick inserted in it comes out dry, about 25 minutes.

Nutrition: Calories: 475 Fat: 38g Carb: 7g Protein: 19g

Easy Bake Keto Bread

Preparation time: 10 minutes

Cooking time: 30 minutes

Servings: 16

Ingredients:

7 whole eggs

4.5 oz. Melted butter

2 tbsp. Warm water

2 tsp dry yeast

1 tsp. Inulin

1 pinch of salt

1 tsp. Xanthan gum

1 tsp. Baking powder

1 tbsp. Psyllium husk powder

2 cups almond flour

Directions:

Preheat the oven to 340f.

In a bowl, mix almond flour, salt, psyllium, baking powder, and xanthan gum.

Make a well in the center of the mixture.

Add the yeast and inulin into the center with the warm water.

Stir the inulin and yeast with the warm water in the center and let the yeast activate, about 10 minutes.

Add in the eggs and melted butter and stir well.

Pour the mixture into a loaf pan lined with parchment paper.

Allow batter to proof in a warm spot covered for 20 minutes with a tea towel.

Place in the oven and bake until golden brown, about 30 to 40 minutes.

Cool, slice, and serve.

Nutrition:

Calories: 140

Fat: 13g

Carb: 3g Protein: 3g

Keto Bakers Bread

Preparation time: 10 minutes

Cooking time: 20 minutes

Servings: 12

Ingredients:

Pinch of salt

4 tbsp. Light cream cheese, softened

½ tsp. Cream of tartar

4 eggs, yolks, and whites separated

Directions:

Heat 2 racks in the middle of the oven at 350f.

Line 2 baking pan with parchment paper, then grease with cooking spray.

Separate egg yolks from the whites and place in separate mixing bowls.

Beat the egg whites and cream of tartar with a hand mixer until stiff, about 3 to 5 minutes. Do not over-beat.

Whisk the cream cheese, salt, and egg yolks until smooth. Slowly fold the cheese mix into the whites until fluffy.

Spoon ¼ cup measure of the batter onto the baking sheets, 6 mounds on each sheet.

Bake in the oven for 20 to 22 minutes, alternating racks halfway through.

Cool and serve.

Nutrition: Calories: 41 Fat: 3.2g Carb: 1g Protein: 2.4g

Keto Cloud Bread Cheese

Preparation time: 5 minutes

Cooking time: 30 minutes

Servings: 12

Ingredients for cream cheese filling:

1 egg yolk

½ tsp. Vanilla stevia drops for filling

8 oz. Softened cream cheese

Base egg dough:

½ tsp. Cream of tartar

1 tbsp. Coconut flour

¼ cup unflavored whey protein

3 oz. Softened cream cheese

¼ tsp. Vanilla stevia drops for dough

4 eggs, separated

Directions:

Preheat the oven to 325f.

Line two baking sheets with parchment paper.

In a bowl, stir the 8 ounces cream cheese, stevia, and egg yolk.

Transfer to the pastry bag.

In another bowl, separate egg yolks from whites.

Add 3 oz. Cream cheese, yolks, stevia, whey protein, and coconut flour. Mix until smooth.

Whip cream of tartar with the egg whites until stiff peaks form.

Fold in the yolk/cream cheese mixture into the beaten whites.

Spoon batter onto each baking sheet, 6 mounds on each. Press each mound to flatten a bit.

Add cream cheese filling in the middle of each batter.

Bake for 30 minutes at 325f.

Nutrition:

Calories: 120

Fat: 10.7g

Carb: 1.1g

Protein: 5.4g

Chapter 7. Lunch

Cauliflower Pizza Crust

Preparation time: 45 minutes

Servings: 1 crust, 8 slices

Directions:

0.5 tsp. Salt

16 oz. Cauliflower florets

1 large egg

1.5 tbsp. Coconut flour

3 tsp. Avocado oil

0.5 tsp. Italian seasoning

1 tsp. Coconut oil

Food blender

Large skillet

Large flat sheet or pizza pan

Directions:

Set your oven to heat at the temperature of 405° fahrenheit.

Pulse the cauliflower in a food blender for approximately 60 seconds until it is a crumbly consistency.

Heat the coconut oil and cauliflower in a frypan for approximately 5 minutes as it becomes tender.

Transfer the cauliflower to a kitchen towel and twist to eliminate the extra water. Repeat this step as many times as necessary to make sure the moisture has been eliminated.

Prepare your pizza pan or flat sheet with of baking lining and set to the side.

In a glass dish, blend the riced cauliflower, salt, egg, coconut flour, avocado oil, and italian seasoning and integrate until it thickens.

Flatten the dough onto the prepped pan to no less than a quarter inch.

Heat for 25 minutes if then and up to half an hour if thicker.

Complete with your favorite toppings and finish in the stove for another 5 minutes. Enjoy!

Expert tip:

For the toppings, be creative with vegetable and meat combinations. The first layer should be your sauce and then layer the meat and vegetables and top with cheese to ensure all ingredients heat properly.

Nutrition:

Protein: 11 grams

Net carbs: 5 grams

Fat: 21 grams

Sugar: 0 grams

Calories: 278

Cauliflower Breakfast Pizza

Servings: 2

Preparation time: 10 minutes

Cooking time: 15 minutes

Ingredients:

2 cups riced cauliflower

4 free range eggs

2 tablespoons coconut flour

1/2 teaspoon kosher salt

1 tablespoon organic psyllium husk powder

Toppings: shredded cooked chicken, sliced avocado, halved cherry tomatoes crumbled goat's cheese

Directions

Start by setting your oven to 350 degrees f. Line your sheet pan with parchment paper.

In a large glass bowl, combine all ingredients until evenly mixed. Let sit for 5 minutes for the dough to thicken and ingredients to marry well.

Spread the dough on the prepared sheet pan and use your hands to shape it into an even pizza crust.

Bake for about 15 minutes, or until golden brown.

Remove from oven and top with toppings. Enjoy!

Nutrition:

Calories: 454; Total fat: 31g; Carbs: 8.8g; Dietary fiber 17.2 g; Protein: 22 g;

Tasty Coconut Pizza Crust

Preparation time: 10 minutes

Cooking time: 25 minutes

Servings: 2

Ingredients

3/4 cup coconut flour sifted

1 teaspoon garlic powder

1 teaspoon apple cider vinegar

3 eggs

3 tablespoons psyllium husk powder

1/2 teaspoon sea salt

1/2 teaspoon baking soda

1 cup boiling hot water

Directions

Set your oven to 350 degrees f and line a baking sheet with parchment paper.

Combine all the dry ingredients in a large mixing bowl. Mix in vinegar and eggs followed by the water and mix until you get a thick, slightly sticky dough.

Wet your hands before spreading out the dough on the baking sheet and bake for 15 minutes or until golden.

Spread your favorite sauce and toppings. Enjoy!

Nutrition: Calories: 189; Total fat: 9g; Carbs: 5.3g; Dietary fiber 8 g; Protein: 7 g;

Mozzarella Pizza Crust

Preparation time: 30 minutes

Servings: 1 crust, 8 slices

Calories: 190

Ingredients:

1.5 cups mozzarella cheese, shredded

0.75 cup almond flour

1 whole egg

2 tbsp. Cream cheese, full-fat

0.25 tsp. Salt

Pizza pan or large flat sheet

Directions:

Set your stove to heat at the temperature of 350° fahrenheit.

Use a microwave-safe dish to nuke the almond flour, mozzarella, and cream cheese for approximately 60 seconds until liquefied.

Toss the cheese and heat for an additional half minute.

Blend the salt and egg into the cheese for about half a minute.

Place a baking lining on the counter and transfer the dough to the middle. Use another baking lining to place on top.

Flatten to no less than a quarter of an inch. Separate the top baking lining and transfer to the pan of choice.

Heat for approximately 13 minutes until turning golden.

Layer with your toppings of choice and heat for about 5 minutes.

Serve hot and enjoy!

Expert tip:

If you have a nut allergy, you can substitute the almond flour with 1/4 cup of coconut flour.

Nutrition:

Protein: 10 grams

Net carbs: 1.4 grams

Fat: 6 grams

Sugar: 2 grams

Herbed Cauliflower Bread

Preparation time: 15 minutes

Cooking time: 45 minutes

Servings: 4

Ingredients

3 cups riced cauliflower

10 free range eggs, separated

1 1/4 cups sifted coconut flour

1 1/2 tablespoons baking powder

6 tablespoons coconut oil or grass-fed butter, melted

6 cloves garlic (minced)

1 tablespoon freshly chopped rosemary

1 tablespoon freshly chopped parsley

1 pinch cream of tartar

Directions

Preheat your oven to 350 degrees f and line a large loaf pan with parchment paper.

Pop the cauliflower in the microwave to steam for 3 minutes then set aside to cool slightly so it is easy to handle.

Combine the egg whites and cream of tartar using a hand mixer until it form firm peaks.

Add a quarter of the stiff egg whites baking powder coconut flour coconut oil or butter, coconut flour and garlic to a food processor and pulse until well combined.

Squeeze excess water from the cauliflower by wrapping it in a cheesecloth and squeezing until dry. Go for as dry as possible. Add this to the food processor and pulse until you get a crumbly mixture and transfer to a mixing bowl.

Fold in the remaining egg whites until well incorporated then fold in the remaining herbs, careful not to over mix.

Scoop the dough into the prepared pan and use the back of a serving spoon to smooth the top. Sprinkle with more herbs, lightly pressing into the dough, if desired and put in the oven to bake for about 45 minutes or until golden and an inserted toothpick comes out clean.

Remove from oven and let cool completely before you slice. Enjoy!

Nutrition: Calories: 269; Total fat: 13g; Carbs: 6.7; Dietary fiber 17 g; Protein: 11g;

Zucchini Pizza Crust

Preparation time: 60 minutes

Cooking time: 20 minutes

Servings: 1 crust, 8 slices

Ingredients:

4 cups zucchini, shredded

1 cup almond flour

2.75 tbsp. Coconut flour

4 tbsp. Nutritional yeast

1.33 tbsp. Italian seasoning

0.75 tsp. Salt

3 large eggs

Kitchen grater

Large flat sheet or pizza pan

Directions:

Adjust the temperature of your stove to heat at 400° fahrenheit.

Cover the desired pan with a layer of baking lining and set to the side.

Use a kitchen grater to shred the zucchini using the largest holes available.

Transfer to a kitchen towel and wring to release all excess moisture.

In a glass dish, blend the coconut flour, zucchini, salt, italian seasoning, nutritional yeast, eggs, and almond flour until integrated and thickened.

Distribute to the prepped sheet and flatten to no less than quarter an inch by hand.

Heat for the duration of 20 minutes. Turn the crust over and warm for another 10 minutes.

Layer with your preferred toppings and heat for another 13 minutes.

Wait about 10 minutes before slicing and serving. Enjoy!

Nutrition: Protein: 7 grams Net carbs: 4 grams Fat: 8 grams Sugar: 1 gram Calories: 127

Fluffy Almond Tortillas

Preparation time: 10 minutes

Cooking time: 5 minutes

Serving: 8

Ingredients

100 g unblanched almond flour

2 teaspoons xanthan gum

25 g coconut flour

1 teaspoon baking powder

1/4 teaspoon sea salt

1 egg lightly beaten

2 teaspoons apple cider vinegar

3 teaspoons water

Directions

Combine the flours baking powder, xanthan gum and sea salt in a food processor and pulse well until well mixed.

Stream in the vinegar as the processor is running then add the egg, still processing and lastly the water. Pulse until the dough forms a ball and is slightly sticky.

Loosely wrap the dough ball in cling wrap and knead for 3 minutes whilst in the plastic cover then let stand for 10 minutes.

Break down the large ball into 8 mini balls and roll them out in between parchment papers until you achieve desired thinness.

Place a non-stick pan over medium heat and let heat up to the point when you pour a few drops of water in the pan, they run through but not too hot that they evaporate.

Cook the tortillas for 5-10 seconds, strictly on each side, this allows them to puff up. Continue cooking until lightly golden.

Best enjoyed hot!

Nutrition:

Calories: 89;

Total fat: 6g;

Carbs: 2g;

Dietary fiber 2 g;

Protein: 3g;

Soft Veggie Tortillas

Preparation time: 30 minutes

Cooking time: 20 minutes

Servings: 3

Ingredients

2 cups freshly riced cauliflower

1/4 cup chopped fresh cilantro

2 large eggs

1/2 lemon, juiced and finely zested

Sea salt & pepper, to taste

Direction

Preheat your oven to 375 degrees f, and use a non-stick baking sheet or line your baking sheet with parchment paper.

Microwave the cauliflower for 3 minutes then set aside to cool slightly. Transfer to a cheesecloth and squeeze out the water until dry then set aside.

In a medium bowl, lightly whisk the eggs. Add in, cilantro, lemon juice and zest cauliflower salt and pepper. Mix until well combined and form 6 small balls. Use your hands to gently shape 6 small "tortillas" on the parchment paper.

Put in the oven and bake for 10 minutes, carefully flip each tortilla, and return to the oven for an additional 5 to 7 minutes, or until completely set and golden.

For additional browning, let the tortillas cool completely then place a small skillet over medium heat. Brown the tortillas, one at a time for 1 minute per side or until browned to desire. Do this for all the tortillas.

Nutrition:

Calories: 37;

Total fat: 1g;

Carbs: 2g;

Dietary fiber 1 g;

Protein: 3g;

Cholesterol:

Keto Butter Flatbread

Preparation time: 5 minutes

Cooking time: 10 minutes

Servings: 4

Ingredients

1 cup blanched almond flour

1 egg + 1 egg white

2 tablespoons coconut flour

½ tsp. Baking powder

2 teaspoons xanthan gum

Falk salt, to taste

1 egg + 1 egg white

2 tablespoons oil for frying

1 tablespoon melted butter

1 tablespoon water

Directions

Combine all the dry ingredients in a mixing bell and mix well.

Whisk in the eggs until well incorporated into the flour.

Wet your hands and add in the tablespoon of water. Knead the dough until it becomes elastic. Divide the dough into 4 parts and wrap each with cling wrap. Let sit for 10 minutes before gently rolling out each ball to form a flat circle. Alternatively, you can press out each ball with your hands.

Place a non-stick pan over medium heat and pour in a quarter of the oil. Cook one flat bread for one minute per side, applying oil on the other side after turning it, and transfer to a hot plate. Repeat for the remaining flat breads.

Once ready, spread the butter (while hot) and top with salt and chopped parsley.

Nutrition:

Calories: 232;

Total fat: 19 g;

Carbs: 9g;

Dietary fiber 9 g;

Protein: 5g;

Tasty Keto Drop Biscuits

Preparation time: 10 minutes

Cooking time: 20 minutes

Servings: 3

Ingredients

1 egg

100 g coconut cream + 2 tsp. Apple cider vinegar, at room temp

2 tablespoons water

100 g almond flour

2 tablespoons coconut flour

2 tablespoons whey protein isolate or more almond flour

1 tablespoon apple cider vinegar

3 1/2 teaspoons baking powder

1 tablespoon flaxseed meal

75 g golden flaxseed meal or psyllium husk, finely ground

1/2 teaspoon kosher salt

7 tablespoons ghee/coconut oil

Directions

Preheat oven to 450 degrees f land line your baking tray with parchment paper or a baking mat.

Whisk together the egg, coconut cream, water and apple cider vinegar in a mixing bowl until very well combined and set aside.

Stir the dry ingredients until well combined. You can use an electric mixer if you find this too cumbersome. Pour in the wet ingredients and continue pulsing. Add the ghee or coconut oil and pulse until well combined but sticky.

Drop small rounds of dough using a serving spoon or tablespoon onto the prepared tray. Lightly brush with ghee and bake for about 15-20 minutes or until browned to desire.

Remove from oven and let cool for 10 minutes before serving.

Nutrition:

Calories: 290;

Total fat: 30 g;

Carbs: 8g;

Dietary fiber 5 g;

Protein: 7g;

Soft Rosemary-Infused Bagels

Preparation time: 5 minutes

Cooking time: 50 minutes

Servings: 4

Ingredients:

1 1/2 cups coconut flour

3/4 teaspoon baking soda

3/4 teaspoon xanthan gum

1/4 teaspoon salt

3 tablespoons ground flaxseed

1 egg

3 egg whites

1/2 cup warm water

1 tablespoon fresh rosemary, finely chopped

Avocado oil

Directions

Set your oven to 250 degrees f.

Mix all the dry ingredients apart from ground flaxseed in a bowl.

Whisk eggs and warm water in a separate bowl. Stir in ground flaxseed until there are no clumps.

Add the egg mixture to the dry ingredients and knead until the dough becomes elastic. Shape it into a bagel and coat with avocado oil.

Press dough into a silicon mold and lightly press the chopped rosemary on top.

Bake in the heated oven for 40 to 50 minutes or until browned to desire.

Nutrition:

Calories: 285;

Total fat: 22.5 g;

Carbs: 12g;

Dietary fiber 7.5 g;

Protein: 13g;

Fluffy Turmeric Veggie Buns

Preparation time: 30 minutes

Cooking time: 30 minutes

Servings: 4

Ingredients

2 cups fresh riced cauliflower

2 free range eggs

2 tablespoons almond flour

2 tablespoons olive oil

¼ teaspoon ground turmeric

Kosher salt and freshly ground pepper to taste

Directions

Preheat your oven to 400 degrees and line a baking sheet with parchment paper or use a non-stick one.

Microwave the cauliflower for 3 minutes then set aside to cool slightly. Transfer to a cheesecloth and squeeze out the water until dry then set aside in a large mixing bowl. Whisk in the eggs, oil, salt, pepper and turmeric.

You can use your hands at this point. Once mixed well, form 6 buns and arrange them on the prepared sheet and bake for about half an hour or until golden.

Serve hot!

Nutrition: Calories: 221; Total fat: 9.3 g;

Carbs: 8g;

Dietary fiber 6 g;

Protein: 8g;

Spicy "Cornbread" Muffins

Preparation time: 10 minutes

Cooking time: 30 minutes

Servings: 12 muffins

Ingredients

1 cup organic coconut flour

1 tbsp. Baking powder

1/3 cup swerve sweetener

1 cup fresh cranberries, halved

Kosher salt, to taste

7 eggs, lightly whisked

1 cup organic almond milk, unsweetened

1/2 cup avocado oil

1/2 tsp. Pure vanilla extract

3 tbsp. Finely chopped jalapeño peppers

1 jalapeño, sliced with seeds removed to garnish

Preheat your oven to 325 degrees f and line a muffin tin with cupcake paper liners.

Combine the dry ingredients using a fork to break up any lumps.

Whisk in the eggs, almond milk and avocado oil. Stir in the vanilla and fold in the chopped pepper and cranberries.

Scoop the batter evenly into the prepared muffin cups and place one slice of jalapeño on top of each.

Bake for 30 minutes or until tops are set and a toothpick inserted in the center comes out clean. Remove from oven and let cool 10 minutes in pan, then remove and let cool completely.

Nutrition: Calories: 157; Total fat: 11.2 g; Carbs: 7.08g; Dietary Fiber 3.84g;

Almond- Cranberry Bread

Preparation time: 10 minutes

Cooking time: i hour 15 minutes

Servings: 6

Ingredients

2 cups blanched almond flour

1 1/2 teaspoons baking powder

1/2 cup swerve sweetener

1/2 teaspoon stevia powder

1/2 teaspoon baking soda

Kosher salt, to taste

4 tablespoons coconut oil

4 free range eggs at room temperature

1/2 cup unsweetened almond milk

1 cup cranberries

Directions

Start by preheating your oven to 350 degrees and line a 9-by-5 inch loaf pan with parchment paper and set aside.

In a large bowl, whisk together all the dry ingredients and set aside.

In a separate bowl, combine the wet ingredients. Pour in the dry ingredients into the wet ingredients until well mixed but not over-mixed. Gently fold in the cranberries then scoop the batter into the prepared tin then transfer to an oven.

Bake for about 1 hour and 15 minutes or until an inserted toothpick comes out clean. Transfer pan and let cool 15 minutes before removing from pan.

Nutrition:

Calories: 179;

Total fat: 15 g;

Carbs: 7g;

Dietary fiber 2g;

Protein: 5.21g;

Itsy Bitsy Pizza Crusts

Preparation time: 10 minutes

Cooking time: 10 minutes

Servings: 2

Ingredients

5 whole eggs and 3 egg whites

1/2 tsp. Baking powder

1/4 cup coconut flour sifted, with more for dusting

Salt, pepper, italian spices

For the sauce:

2 garlic cloves, minced

1/2 cup organic tomato sauce

1 tsp. Dried basil

1/4 tsp. Pink sea salt

Directions

Star by whisking the eggs and egg whites until opaque in a mixing bowl. Whisk in the coconut flour until all clumps are removed then add all the remaining ingredients and continue whisking until well combined.

Lightly grease a small pan and place over medium-low heat. Pour some of the batter evenly once the pan is hot. Cover and let cook for about 3-5minutes or until bubbles form on top. Flip the other side and cook for 2 minutes.

Transfer to a platter and repeat this for the remaining batter. Once the crusts are cool, use a fork to roughly poke holes on the crusts. This will help them cook evenly. Lightly dust with coconut flour and set aside.

For the sauce, whisk all the ingredients together then let stand for 30 minutes to allow thickening.

Spread the pizza bases with the sauce and top with your favorite toppings and bake for about 3-5 minutes or until done to desire.

Nutrition:

Calories: 125;

Total fat: 1 g;

Carbs: 6;

Dietary fiber 3g;

Protein: 8g;

Chapter 8. Dinner

Low Carb Yeast Bread

Preparation time: 10 minutes

Cooking time: 4 hours

Servings: 16 slices

Ingredients

1 teaspoon salt

4 tablespoons oat flour

1 package dry yeast rapid rise/highly active

1 1/2 teaspoons baking powder

1/2 teaspoon sugar

1 1/8 cups warm water

1/4 cup coarse unprocessed wheat bran

3 tablespoons olive oil

1/4 cup flax meal

1 cup vital wheat gluten flour

3/4 cup soy flour

Directions:

Add water, yeast and sugar to the bread machine and let rest there for 10 minutes.

Add the remaining ingredients and select bread mode on the machine.

After the cooking time is over, remove the bread from the machine and let rest for about 10 minutes. Enjoy!

Nutrition:

99 calories;

5 g fat;

7 g total carbs;

9 g protein

Keto Sandwich Bread

Preparation time: 10 minutes

Cooking time: 25 minutes

Servings: 12 slices

Ingredients

1 tablespoon xantham gum

1 1/4 cups warm water

2 1/2 cups almond flour

1/2 teaspoon salt

2 cups whey protein

3 teaspoons baking powder

Directions:

Add all ingredients to the bread machine.

Select dough setting and press start. Mix ingredients for about 4-5 minutes. After that press stop button.

Smooth out the top of the loaf. Choose bake mode and press start. Cook for about 20-25 minutes and press stop.

Let the bread rest for about 10 minutes. Enjoy!

Nutrition: 197 calories; 12 g fat; 8 g total carbs; 18 g protein

Seeded Bread

Preparation time: 10 minutes

Cooking time: 40 minutes

Servings: 16 slices

Ingredients

2 tablespoons chia seeds

1/4 teaspoon salt

7 large eggs

1/2 teaspoon xanthan gum

2 cups almond flour

1 teaspoon baking powder

1/2 cup unsalted butter

3 tablespoons sesame seeds

2 tablespoons olive oil

Directions:

Add all the ingredients to the bread machine.

Close the lid and choose bread mode. Once done, take out from machine and cut into at least 16 slices.

This keto seeded bread can be kept for up to 4-5 days in the fridge.

Nutrition: 101 calories; 16 g fat; 4 g total carbs; 6 g protein

Cinnamon Sweet Bread

Preparation time: 10 minutes

Cooking time: 1 hour

Servings: 12

Ingredients

3 teaspoons ground cinnamon

1 ½ cups of almond flour

3 large eggs

½ cup keto sweetener

1 teaspoon vanilla essence

¼ cup coconut flour

¼ cup sour cream

1 teaspoon baking powder

½ cup unsweetened almond milk

½ cup unsalted butter, melted

Directions:

Add all ingredients to the bread machine.

Close the lid and choose the sweet bread mode.

After the cooking time is over, remove the bread from the machine and let rest for about 10 minutes.
Enjoy!

Nutrition: 191 calories; 17 g fat; 5 g total carbs; 5 g protein

Nut And Seed Bread

Cooking time: 45 minutes

Servings: 16 slices

Ingredients

1 cup pumpkin seeds

1 teaspoon salt

1/2 cup almond flour

4 eggs, whisked

1/2 cup whole almonds

1 tablespoon lemon juice

1 cup raw pecans

¼ cup olive oil

1/2 cup hazelnuts

1/4 cup poppy seeds

1/2 cup flax meal

1 cup sunflower seeds

1/2 cup chia seeds

Directions:

Add all the ingredients to the bread machine.

Close the lid and choose bread mode. Once done, take out from machine and cut into at least 16 slices.

Nutrition:

316 calories;

28 g fat;

11 g total carbs;

11 g protein

Gluten Free Keto Tortillas

Preparation time: 10 minutes

Cooking time: 5 minutes

Servings: 8

Ingredients

1 teaspoon baking powder

3 teaspoons water

¼ cup almond flour

1 egg, lightly beaten

2 tablespoons coconut flour

2 teaspoons apple cider vinegar

2 teaspoons xanthan gum

1/4 teaspoon kosher salt

Directions:

Add all ingredients to the bread machine.

Select dough setting and press start. Mix ingredients for about 4-5 minutes. After that press stop button.

When the time is over, transfer the dough to the floured surface. Shape it into a ball and then cut into even pieces. Roll the pieces out into tortillas.

Preheat a pan/skillet over medium-high heat.

Cook tortillas over medium heat until each side becomes light golden brown, for about 30-40 seconds.

Once done, take out from the skillet. Serve warm and enjoy!

Nutrition:

89 calories;

6 g fat; 4 g total carbs; 3 g protein

Almond Bread Loaf

Preparation time: 10 minutes

Cooking time: 3 hours 22 minutes

Servings: 15

Ingredients:

2 ½ cups almond flour

1/3 cup coconut flour

½ teaspoon xanthan gum

1 ½ teaspoons baking powder

¼ teaspoon salt

Sesame seeds

¼ cup butter, melted and cooled

5 eggs

2/3 cup almond milk

¼ teaspoon tartar cream

Directions:

Add all the ingredients to the bread machine.

Close the lid and choose bread mode. Once done, take out from machine and cut into at least 16 slices.

Nutrition: 215 calories, 10.1g fat, 5g total carbs, 25.2g protein

Sugar Free Banana Bread

Preparation time: 10 minutes

Cooking time: 3 hours 18 minutes

Servings: 8

Ingredients:

1 ½ cups almond flour

¼ cup granulated erythritol sweetener

1 teaspoon baking powder

2 teaspoons cinnamon

¼ cup walnuts, crushed

½ cup banana, mashed

2 tablespoons butter, melted

3 eggs

Directions:

Add all ingredients to the bread machine.

Close the lid and choose the sweet bread mode.

After the cooking time is over, remove the bread from the machine and let rest for about 10 minutes. Enjoy!

Nutrition: 205 calories, 17.2g fat, 6.4g total carbs, 8g protein

Collagen Bread

Preparation time: 10 minutes

Cooking time: 3 hours 22 minutes

Servings: 12

Ingredients:

6 tablespoons almond flour

½ cup collagen protein, unflavored

1 teaspoon baking powder

1 teaspoon xanthan gum

Pinch of pink salt

5 eggs, separated

1 tablespoon coconut oil, unflavored and liquid

Directions:

Add all the ingredients to the bread machine.

Close the lid and choose bread mode. Once done, take out from machine and cut into at least 16 slices.

Nutrition:

77 calories,

5g fat,

1g total carbs,

7g protein

Macadamia Bread

Preparation time: 10 minutes

Cooking time: 60 minutes

Servings: 8

Ingredients:

¼ cup almond flour

1 cup macadamia nuts

2 tablespoons flax meal

1 teaspoon baking powder

2 scoops whey protein powder

4 eggs

2 egg whites

1 tablespoon lemon juice

¼ cup butter, melted

Directions:

Add all the ingredients to the bread machine.

Close the lid and choose express bake mode. Once done, take out from machine and cut into at least 16 slices.

Nutrition: 257 calories, 22.4g fat, 4.5g total carbs, 11.5g protein

Blueberry Bread

Preparation time: 10 minutes

Cooking time: 3 hours 18 minutes

Servings: 12

Ingredients:

2 tablespoons coconut flour

2 cups almond flour

1 ½ teaspoons baking powder

½ cup erythritol sweetener

5 eggs

½ cup blueberries

3 tablespoons heavy whipping cream

3 tablespoons butter, softened

1 teaspoon vanilla extract

Directions:

Add all ingredients to the bread machine.

Close the lid and choose the sweet bread mode.

After the cooking time is over, remove the bread from the machine and let rest for about 10 minutes. Enjoy!

Nutrition: 175 calories, 15g fat, 3g total carbs, 6g protein

Pumpkin bread

Preparation time: 10 minutes

Cooking time: 70 minutes

Servings: 12

Ingredients:

1 ½ teaspoons baking powder

2 teaspoons cinnamon powder

1 ½ cups almond flour, milled

1 tablespoon psyllium husk powder

½ cup golden flax meal

1 ½ teaspoons ground ginger

¼ teaspoon ground cloves

¼ cup walnuts, chopped

½ teaspoon ground nutmeg

½ cup confectioner's erythritol

4 eggs

7 oz. Pumpkin puree, canned

1 cup granulated sugar substitute

1 teaspoon vanilla extract

¼ cup + 2 tablespoons butter, melted

4 oz. Full-fat cream cheese, softened

2 tablespoons heavy whipping cream

Directions:

Add all ingredients to the bread machine.

Select dough setting and press start. Mix ingredients for about 4-5 minutes. After that press stop button.

Smooth out the top of the loaf. Choose bake mode and press start. Cook for about 50-55 minutes and press stop.

Let the bread rest for about 10 minutes. Enjoy!

Nutrition: 225 calories, 15.8g fat, 4.9g total carbs, 6.4g protein

Zucchini Chocolate Bread

Preparation time: 10 minutes

Cooking time: 45 minutes

Servings: 12

Ingredients:

1 ¼ cups almond flour

½ teaspoon baking soda

¼ cup cocoa powder

1 teaspoon baking powder

A pinch of salt

3 eggs

½ teaspoon stevia

2 tablespoons coconut oil

1 cup zucchini, grated

Directions:

Add all ingredients to the bread machine. Select dough setting and press start. Mix ingredients for about 4-5 minutes. After that press stop button.

Smooth out the top of the loaf. Choose bake mode and press start. Cook for about 40-45 minutes and press stop.

Let the bread rest for about 10 minutes. Enjoy!

Nutrition: 57 calories, 5g fat, 1g total carbs, 3g protein

Yeasted Avocado Bread

Preparation time: 10 minutes

Cooking time: 3 hours 22 minutes

Servings: 10

Ingredients:

2 + ½ teaspoon active dry yeast

1 teaspoon erythritol

2 teaspoons baking powder

1/3 cup golden flax meal

½ cup almond flour

¼ cup whole psyllium husk

1 teaspoon sea salt

½ cup hot water

4 eggs

1 avocado

¼ cup extra water

2 tablespoons olive oil

Directions:

Add water, yeast and erythritol to the bread machine and let rest there for 10 minutes.

Add the remaining ingredients and select bread mode on the machine.

After the cooking time is over, remove the bread from the machine and let rest for about 10 minutes. Enjoy!

Nutrition:

101 calories,

8.3g fat,

3g total carbs,

4g protein

Coconut Bread

Preparation time: 10 minutes

Cooking time: 60 minutes

Servings: 10

Ingredients:

½ cup coconut flour

¼ teaspoon baking soda

¼ teaspoon salt

6 eggs

¼ cup coconut oil, melted

¼ cup almond milk, unsweetened

Directions:

Add all ingredients to the bread machine.

Select dough setting and press start. Mix ingredients for about 4-5 minutes. After that press stop button.

Smooth out the top of the loaf. Choose bake mode and press start. Cook for about 50-55 minutes and press stop.

Let the bread rest for about 10 minutes. Enjoy!

Nutrition: 108 calories, 8.7g fat, 3.4g total carbs, 4.2g protein

Orangey Almond Bacon Bread

Preparation time: 10 minutes

Cooking time: 3 hours 18 minutes

Servings: 10

Ingredients

1 ½ cups almond flour

1 tablespoon baking powder

7 oz bacon, diced

2 eggs

1 ½ cups cheddar cheese, shredded

4 tablespoons butter, melted

1/3 cup sour cream

Directions:

Add all ingredients to the bread machine.

Close the lid and choose the sweet bread mode.

After the cooking time is over, remove the bread from the machine and let rest for about 10 minutes. Enjoy!

Nutrition:

307 calories,

26 g fat,

3 g total carbs,

14 g protein

Cranberry Bread

Preparation time: 10 minutes

Cooking time: 3 hours 18 minutes

Servings: 12

Ingredients

2 ½ cups almond flour

2 teaspoon baking powder

2 cups fresh cranberries

1 tablespoon orange zest

1 cup erythritol or stevia

½ teaspoon salt

8 eggs

8 oz cream cheese

2 teaspoons orange extract

½ cup unsalted butter

Directions:

Add all ingredients to the bread machine.

Close the lid and choose the sweet bread mode.

After the cooking time is over, remove the bread from the machine and let rest for about 10 minutes. Enjoy!

Nutrition: 337 calories, 31 g fat, 7 g total carbs, 10 g protein

Cheesy Bread With Herbs

Preparation time: 10 minutes

Cooking time: 45 minutes

Servings: 12

Ingredients

2 cups almond flour

1 teaspoon baking powder

½ teaspoon xantham gum

1 tablespoon dried parsley

½ tablespoon dried oregano

2 tablespoons garlic powder

½ teaspoon salt

1 cup cheddar cheese, shredded

6 eggs, beaten

½ cup butter, softened

Directions:

Add all ingredients to the bread machine.

Select dough setting and press start. Mix ingredients for about 4-5 minutes. After that press stop button.

Smooth out the top of the loaf. Choose bake mode and press start. Cook for about 45-50 minutes and press stop.

Let the bread rest for about 10 minutes. Enjoy!

Nutrition:

154 calories,

13.4 g fat,

3 g total carbs,

6 g protein

Lemon Bread

Preparation time: 10 minutes

Cooking time: 3 hours 18 minutes

Servings: 16

Ingredients

2 cups almond flour

¼ cup coconut flour

1 tablespoon baking powder

¾ cup xylitol

5 eggs

½ cup butter, melted

¼ cup lemon juice

For the glaze:

2 tablespoons lemon juice

1 cup powdered erythritol

Directions:

Add all ingredients to the bread machine. Close the lid and choose the sweet bread mode. After the cooking time is over, remove the bread from the machine and let it cool.

Combine lemon juice and erythritol in a bowl until well mixed. Drizzle lemon glazing all over the top. Slice and serve.

Nutrition: 174 calories, 11 g fat, 5 g total carbs, 4 g protein

Pull-Apart Bread Rolls

Preparation time: 10 minutes

Cooking time: 15 minutes + dough preparation

Servings: 8

Ingredients:

2 cups almond flour

3 tablespoons psyllium husk powder

2 teaspoons baking powder

3 tablespoons whey protein powder

2 teaspoons insulin

2 teaspoons active dry yeast

2 egg whites

2 eggs

¼ cup butter

1/3 cup lukewarm water

¼ cup greek yoghurt

Directions:

Add all ingredients to the bread machine.

Select dough setting. When the time is over, transfer the dough to the floured surface. Shape it into a ball and then cut into about 8 even pieces.

Line a pie dish with parchment paper. Form 8 dough balls. Cover the dish with greased cling film and let sit for 60 minutes in a warm place.

Heat the oven to 350f and bake for 15 minutes. Cover with foil and bake for 10 more minutes.

Nutrition:

257 calories,

20.1g fat,

7.1g total carbs,

12.4g protein

Cinnamon Roll Knots

Preparation time: 10 minutes

Cooking time: 20 minutes + dough preparation

Servings: 10

Ingredients:

1 cup almond flour

¼ cup coconut flour

2 teaspoons baking powder

2 teaspoons xanthan gum

4 tablespoons golden erythritol sweetener

2 teaspoons cinnamon

¼ teaspoon salt

2 teaspoons apple cider vinegar

1 egg

5 teaspoons water

1 tablespoon butter

Directions:

Add all ingredients to the bread machine.

Select dough setting. When the time is over, transfer the dough to the floured surface. Shape it into a ball.

Line a baking dish with parchment paper and roll the dough on the lined baking sheet. Brush with melted butter and add cinnamon. Fold dough balls in half and cut into 10 strips. Twist and form knots and make seal closed.

Heat the oven to 350f, add knots to the baking dish and bake for 20 minutes.

Nutrition:

40 calories,

3.5g fat,

2g total carbs,

2g protein

Rosemary Garlic Dinner Rolls

Preparation time: 10 minutes

Cooking time: 30 minutes

Servings: 10

Ingredients:

½ teaspoon baking powder

1/3 cup ground flax seed

1 cup mozzarella cheese, shredded

1 cup almond flour

1 teaspoon rosemary, minced

A pinch of salt

1 oz. Cream cheese

1 egg, beaten

1 tablespoon butter

1 teaspoon garlic, minced

Directions:

Add all ingredients to the bread machine.

Select dough setting. When the time is over, transfer the dough to the floured surface. Shape it into a ball.

Roll the dough into a log and slice into 6 slices. Place on a greased baking sheet.

Combine rosemary, garlic and butter in a bowl and mix. Brush half of this over the biscuits.

Heat the oven to 400f and bake for 15 minutes.

Brush with the remaining mixture and add salt before serving.

Nutrition:

168 calories,

12.9g fat,

5.4g total carbs,

10.3g protein

Chapter 9. Snack And Dessert

Strawberry Mascarpone Tart

Preparation time: 10 minutes

Cooking time: 15 minutes

Serving: 12

Ingredients

For the coconut base:

1/2 cup avocado oil

3/4 cup and 2 tablespoons coconut flour

2 eggs, pastured

1 teaspoon vanilla extract, unsweetened

1 teaspoon erythritol sweetener

For the mascarpone cream:

1 cup strawberries

1 teaspoon vanilla extract, unsweetened

2 tablespoons erythritol sweetener

1 cup mascarpone, full-fat

2 eggs, pastured, separated

Directions

Switch on the oven, set it to 356 degrees f and let preheat.

Meanwhile, prepare the base and for this, crack eggs in a bowl, add oil, sweetener, and vanilla and blend using a stick blender until well combined.

Slowly blend in flour until it has incorporated and a sticky dough comes together and refrigerate it for 10 minutes or until cooked.

Then take a large piece of parchment sheet, place the dough on it, cover its top with another parchment sheet, and roll into thin crust.

Take a 9-inches pie pan, grease it with oil, then place curst on it, press it into the pan and bake for 10 minutes or until the edges of pie are lightly browned.

Meanwhile, prepare the cream filling and for this, place egg yolks in a bowl, add mascarpone, sweetener, and vanilla and beat until well combined.

Then beat egg whites in another bowl with a whisker until stiff peaks form and fold in egg yolks until mixed.

When the pie crust has baked, let it cool for 15 minutes, then fill it with mascarpone mixture, smooth the top and chill the pie in the refrigerator for 30 minutes or until cooled.

Top with berries, then cut the pie into slices and serve.

Nutrition:

Cal; 21.5 g

Fats; 4.2 g

 Protein; 3.8 g

Net carb; 3.8 g Fiber; 236

Dark Chocolate Tart

Preparation time: 10 minutes

Cooking time: 15 minutes

Serving: 8

Ingredients

For the crust:

6 tablespoons coconut flour

2 tablespoons erythritol sweetener

4 tablespoons butter, melted

1 egg, pastured

For the filling:

1/4 cup erythritol sweetener

30 drops of liquid stevia

2 ounces chocolate, unsweetened

1 egg, pastured

1/2 cup heavy whipping cream, grass-fed, full-fat

1-ounce cream cheese, full-fat

Directions

Switch on the oven, set it to 350 degrees f and let preheat.

Meanwhile, prepare the crust and for this, place all the ingredients for it in a bowl and stir until well mixed.

Take two 4-inches tart pan, divide the crust mixture in it, then spread it evenly on the bottom and sides of the pan, poke holes in the crust and bake for 10 to 12 minutes or until the edges are nicely golden brown.

Meanwhile, prepare the filling and for this, place a pot over medium heat, add cream and cook for 5 minutes or until thoroughly heated.

Remove the pot from heat, add chocolate into the cream and blend using an immersion blender until well combined.

Then blend in the egg, stevia, erythritol, and cream cheese until smooth and set aside until required.

When the tarts have baked, let them cool for 20 minutes, then evenly pour in prepared filling and bake for 15 minutes at 325 degrees f until done.

When done, let tart cools for 30 minutes at room temperature and then chill in the refrigerator for 2 hours until set.

Serve when ready.

Nutrition:

190 cal;

17.2 g fats;

3 g protein;

1.7 g net carb; 3.8 g fiber;

Toasted Cream Tarts

Preparation time: 10 minutes

Cooking time: 15 minutes

Serving: 24

Ingredients

For toasted cream:

1 tablespoon erythritol sweetener

1/4 teaspoon baking soda

1/4 teaspoon cinnamon

2 ¼ cups heavy cream, grass-fed, full-fat

For tart shells:

3/4 cup and 1 tablespoon almond flour, full-fat

1/4 teaspoon cinnamon

1 tablespoon swerve sweetener

1 1/2 cups shredded mozzarella cheese

1 egg, pastured

1 tablespoon cream cheese, full-fat

Directions

Prepare the toasted cream and for this, pour cream in a large bowl, add baking soda, stir well until mixed, then evenly divide the mixture into three mason jars and secure them with lid.

Switch on the instant pot, pour in 1-inch water, then insert a steamer rack in it and place mason jars on it.

Shut the instant pot with its lid, cook at high pressure for 2 hours and when done, do natural pressure release.

Let the mason jars cool into the instant pot until cool enough to handle, then take them out and refrigerate until chilled.

Then set the oven to 400 degrees f and let preheat.

Meanwhile, prepare the tart shells and for this, place cream cheese and mozzarella cheese in a heatproof bowl and microwave for 1 minute until cheese melts, stirring halfway through.

Let melted cheese rest for 5 minutes, add cinnamon, sweetener, egg, and flour, stir until incorporated and the dough comes together and then roll the dough into thin crust between two parchment sheets.

Remove the top parchment sheet and then cut out mini muffin holes by using a cookie cutter.

Take a muffin tray, grease it with oil, place a muffin dough hole into a muffin cup and press by using fingertips.

Place the muffin tray into the oven to bake tarts for 12 to 15 minutes and then let them cool on a wire rack.

Then take out the chilled cream, pour it in a bowl, add sweetener and whip until well combined. Spoon the cream in a piping bag, then fill the cool tarts with it and dust with cinnamon. Serve straight away.

Nutrition: 124 cal; 11.7 g fats; 3.1 g protein; 1.3 g net carb; 0.4 g fiber;

Rhubarb Tart

Preparation time: 10 minutes

Cooking time: 15 minutes

Serving: 8

Ingredients

For the crust:

6 ounces almond flour

¾ ounces shredded coconut, unsweetened

1/3 cup erythritol sweetener

3 ounces butter, unsalted

For the almond cream filling:

1¾ cups almond flour

7 ounces rhubarb

½ cup erythritol sweetener

4¼ ounces butter, unsalted, softened

1 teaspoon vanilla extract, unsweetened

3 eggs, pastured

Directions

Switch on the oven, set it to 360 degrees f and let preheat.

Meanwhile, prepare the crust and for this, place flour in a bowl, add coconut and sweetener and stir until combined.

Place butter in a heatproof bowl, microwave for 1 minute or until it melts, then add it into the flour mixture and mix well until the dough comes together.

Take a 9-inches tart pan, grease it with oil, place the dough on it and spread it evenly in the bottom and sides of the pan.

Bake the crust for 10 minutes or until nicely golden brown and then let cool for 10 minutes.

Meanwhile, prepare the cream filling and for this, place the butter in a bowl add sweetener and beat until fluffy.

Then beat in eggs, vanilla and almond flour in batches until smooth and then set aside until required.

When the tart has baked, take it out and fill it with prepared creamy filling.

Peel rhubarb stalks by using a vegetable peeler, add into the filling, and then push the rhubarb peels firmly.

Bake the tart for another 35 minutes or until set, then let cool at room temperature for 10 minutes, chill in the refrigerator until cooled and then slice to serve.

Nutrition:

515 cal;

49 g fats;

11 g protein;

2 g net carb; 1 g fiber;

Lemon Curd Tart

Preparation time: 10 minutes

Cooking time: 15 minutes

Serving: 12

Ingredients

1 cup lemon curd, full-fat, chilled

12 ounces fresh blackberries

1 tablespoon sliced almonds

For the crust: 1 ½ cup almond flour - 1/2 cup coconut flour

4 tablespoons erythritol sweetener, powdered - 2 eggs, pastured

4 tablespoons unsalted butter, cold

Directions

Set oven to 350 degrees f and set aside until required. Prepare the pie crust, and for this, place all its ingredients in a large bowl, stir until well mixed, then shape the mixture into a dough ball and divide it into two. Take two tart pans, grease them with oil, line the pans with parchment sheet, then add a dough into each tart pan and spread evenly in the bottom and sides of the pan.

Bake the tarts for 15 minutes until nicely golden brown and then thoroughly cooled. Then take out the tart crust, place them in a dish, fill evenly with lemon curd, and cover the top with berries. Sprinkle almonds on berries and serve straight away.

Nutrition: 216 cal; 20 g fats; 7.8 g protein; 10.6 g net carb; 5.7 g fiber;

Strawberry Cheesecake Tarts

Preparation time: 10 minutes

Cooking time: 15 minutes

Serving: 4

Ingredients

For the crust:

3 ounces butter, unsalted, melted

1/4 cup and 1 tablespoon erythritol sweetener

2 cups almond flour

For the cheesecake filling:

1/4 cup and 1 tablespoon confectioners erythritol sweetener

1/2 teaspoon vanilla extract, unsweetened

1 cup cream cheese, full-fat

1/2 cup heavy whipping cream, grass-fed, full-fat

For the berry topping:

1 cup strawberries, fresh

1/4 teaspoon vanilla extract, unsweetened

1 teaspoon erythritol sweetener

Directions

Switch on the oven, set it to 350 degrees f and let preheat.

Meanwhile, prepare the crust and for this, place almond flour in a bowl, add butter and sweetener, then stir well until incorporated and the dough comes together and divide the dough into six.

Then take four 5-inches tart pans, place a dough in each pan, spread it evenly in the bottom and sides of the pan and then prick the crusts with a fork.

Bake the tarts for 15 minutes or until nicely golden brown and then cool for 30 minutes.

Meanwhile, prepare the berry topping and for this, cut the berries into the quarter, then place them in a bowl, sprinkle with sweetener, drizzle with vanilla and stir until well coated.

Take a baking tray, line it with parchment sheet, spread the berries on it in a single layer and bake for 15 to 20 minutes or until softened, let cool until required.

While berries are baking, prepare the cheesecake filling and for this, beat cream cheese, vanilla, and sweetener in a bowl until fluffy and then beat in cream until smooth.

Divide the cooled berries in half and then pass the one-half of berries through a fine sieve placed on a bowl until smooth, remove and discard the seeds.

Add one half of the cheesecake filling into pureed berries, reserving 1 tablespoon of pureed berries, then pour the mixture in two tart pans and a smooth the top.

Add remaining cheesecake filling in remaining tart shells, smooth the top, evenly spoon reserved strawberry puree on top and swirl with a toothpick.

Let the tart chill in the refrigerator for 1 hour or until set, then top with remaining roasted berries and serve.

Nutrition:

482 cal; 48 g fats; 10.6 g protein; 7.1 g net carb; 4 g fiber;

Chocolate Tart With Raspberries

Preparation time: 10 minutes

Cooking time: 15 minutes

Serving: 10

Ingredients

For the pie crust:

1 1/3 cups almond flour

3 tablespoons cold butter, unsalted

1 1/2 teaspoon coconut flour

1 ½ teaspoon water, cold

For the ganache:

1/3 cup erythritol sweetener, powdered

4 ounces chocolate chips, unsweetened

4 ounces heavy cream, grass-fed, full-fat

Directions

Switch on the oven, set it to 350 degrees f and let preheat.

Meanwhile, prepare the crust and for this, place all its ingredients in a food processor and pulse until incorporated and the dough comes together.

Transfer the dough in a pie pan, spread it evenly in the bottom and sides, then bake for 14 minutes or until golden brown and let cool completely.

Meanwhile, prepare the cream filling and for this, place the cream in a heatproof bowl and microwave for 2 minutes or until bubbles form around the edges.

Add chocolate into the hot cream, stir until melted, then whisk in sweetener smooth and pour the mixture into the pie crust.

Spread the creamy mixture evenly, smooth the top and chill the tart in the refrigerator for 30 minutes or until set.

Top the tart with berries and serve.

Nutrition:

213 cal;

21 g fats; 5 g protein; 4 g net carb; 3 g fiber;

Blueberry Zucchini Bread

Preparation time: 10 minutes

Cooking time: 15 minutes

Serving: 18

Ingredients

1 cup blueberries

1 1/2 cup grated zucchini, moisture removed

2 cups almond flour, blanched

2 teaspoons baking powder

1/4 teaspoon sea salt

1 teaspoon vanilla extract, unsweetened

3/4 cup erythritol sweetener

1/2 cup butter, unsalted, softened

1 tablespoon lemon juice

1 tablespoon lemon zest

3 eggs, pastured

Directions

Switch on the oven, set it to 325 degrees f and let preheat.

Meanwhile, place butter and sweetener in a bowl, whisk until fluffy and then beat in eggs, lemon zest and juice, vanilla until combined.

Then beat in flour, salt, baking powder until incorporated, fold in zucchini and berries, and stir until well mixed.

Take a 9 by 5 inches loaf pan, line it with parchment paper, spoon in batter and bake the bread for 1 hour and 10 minutes or until the bread has cooked and an inserted knife into the bread comes out clean.

Then let the bread cool in the pan completely, cut into 18 slices, and serve.

Nutrition:

139 cal;

12 g fats;

4 g protein;

3 g net carb;

2 g fiber;

Blueberry Bread

Preparation time: 10 minutes

Cooking time: 15 minutes

Serving: 12

Ingredients

1/2 cup blueberries

2 cups almond flour, blanched

1/2 cup erythritol sweetener

2 tablespoons coconut flour

1 teaspoon vanilla extract, unsweetened

1 1/2 teaspoon baking powder

3 tablespoons butter, unsalted, softened

5 eggs, pastured

3 tablespoons heavy whipping cream, grass-fed, full-fat

Directions

Switch on the oven, set it to 350 degrees f and let preheat.

Meanwhile, add vanilla in a bowl along with sweetener and eggs, whisk using an immersion blender until frothy, and then whisk in the cream until combined.

Place remaining ingredients in another bowl, except for butter and berries, stir until mixed, then slowly mix into egg mixture until incorporated and fold in berries until combined.

Take a 9 by 5 inches loaf pan, grease it with butter, pour in prepared batter and bake for 45 to 50 minutes or until the bread has cooked and an inserted toothpick into the bread comes out clean.

Let bread cool in its pan for 10 minutes, then take it out to cool completely on a wire rack, cut the bread into 12 slices and serve.

Nutrition:

175 cal;

15 g fats; 6 g protein; 3 g net carb; 2 g fiber;

Banana Bread

Preparation time: 10 minutes

Cooking time: 15 minutes

Serving: 12

Ingredients

2 cup almond flour, blanched

1/4 cup coconut flour

1/2 cup walnuts, chopped

1/4 teaspoon sea salt

2 teaspoons baking powder

1/2 cup erythritol sweetener

2 teaspoons cinnamon

2 teaspoons banana extract, unsweetened

6 tablespoons butter, unsalted, softened

4 eggs, pastured

1/4 cup almond milk, full-fat, unsweetened

Directions

Switch on the oven, set it to 350 degrees f and let preheat.

Meanwhile, place flours, salt, baking powder, and cinnamon in a bowl and stir until mixed.

Place butter into another bowl, add sweetener, beat until fluffy and then beat in eggs, banana extract and milk until combined.

Slowly beat in flour mixture until incorporated and a smooth, fold in walnuts and transfer the batter into a 9 by 5 inches loaf pan, lined with parchment sheet.

Bake the bread for 1 hour until the bread has cooked and an inserted toothpick slides out clean.

Let bread cool completely into the pan, then take it out, cut into 12 pieces, and serve.

Nutrition:

224 cal;

20 g fats;

8 g protein;

2 g net carb;

4 g fiber;

Pumpkin Bread

Preparation time: 10 minutes

Cooking time: 15 minutes

Serving: 12

Ingredients

1/2 cup coconut flour

2 cup almond flour, blanched

1/4 teaspoon sea salt

2 teaspoons pumpkin pie spice

1/4 cup pumpkin seeds

2 teaspoons baking powder

3/4 cup erythritol sweetener

1/3 cup avocado oil

3/4 cup pumpkin puree

4 eggs, beaten

Directions

Switch on the oven, set it to 350 degrees f and let preheat.

Meanwhile, place flours in a bowl, stir in sweetener, salt, baking powder, and pumpkin spice, and then whisk in butter, eggs and pumpkin puree until incorporated and a smooth.

Take a 9 by 5 inches loaf pan, pour in batter, smooth the batter from the top, sprinkle pumpkin seeds on top and bake for the bread for 1 hour or until the bread has cooked and an inserted toothpick slides out clean.

Let the bread cool in its pan, then take it out, cut into 12 slices and serve.

Nutrition:

215 cal; 18 g fats; 8 g protein; 4 g net carb; 5 g fiber

Cinnamon Butter Loaf

Preparation time: 10 minutes

Cooking time: 15 minutes

Serving: 16

Ingredients

2 1/2 cups almond flour, blanched

1/4 cup chopped walnuts

4 tablespoons psyllium husk

1/2 teaspoon salt

1 tablespoon and 2 teaspoons cinnamon

1 teaspoon baking powder

1/2 cup erythritol sweetener

1/4 cup avocado oil

1/2 cup hot water

4 eggs, pastured

Directions

Switch on the oven, set it to 375 degrees f and let preheat.

Meanwhile, place flour in a bowl, add husk, salt, sweetener, baking powder, and 1 tablespoon cinnamon until mixed.

Then whisk in hot water, eggs, and oil until combined, take an 8 inches loaf pan, grease it with oil and pour in half of the batter.

Sprinkle with remaining cinnamon, pour in remaining batter, then create patterns into the batter by swirling it with a knife and top with walnuts.

Bake the bread for 40 minutes or until the bread has cooked and an inserted skewer into the pan slides out clean.

Let the bread cool in the pan, then take it out, cut into 16 slices, and serve.

Nutrition:

166 cal;

14 g fats;

5 g protein;

3 g net carb;

4 g fiber;

Cinnamon Bread

Preparation time: 10 minutes

Cooking time: 15 minutes

Serving: 12

Ingredients

2 cups almond flour

1 teaspoon baking soda

⅓ cup erythritol sweetener

1 teaspoon baking powder

2 tablespoons cinnamon

2 teaspoons vanilla extract, unsweetened

¼ cup melted butter

3 tablespoons sour cream, full-fat

3 eggs, pastured

Directions

Switch on the oven, set it to 350 degrees f and let preheat.

Meanwhile, place butter and sweetener in a bowl, beat until fluffy, and then beat in cream, vanilla, and eggs until well combined.

Stir together flour, baking soda, baking powder and cinnamon in another bowl, and then slowly beat into egg mixture until smooth and incorporated.

Take a loaf pan, grease it with oil, pour in the batter and bake for 30 to 40 minutes until done and an inserted skewer into the bread slides out clean.

Let the bread cool in the pan, then take it out, cut into 12 slices, and serve.

Nutrition:

200 cal;

18 g fats;

7 g protein;

4 g net carb;

3 g fiber;

Macadamia Nut Bread

Preparation time: 15 minutes

Cooking time: 25 minutes

Serving: 10

Ingredients

1/4 cup coconut flour

5 ounces macadamia nuts

5 eggs, pastured

1/2 teaspoon baking soda

1/2 teaspoon apple cider vinegar

Directions

Switch on the oven, set it to 350 degrees f and let preheat.

Meanwhile, add nuts in a food processor, blend until nut butter comes together and then blend in eggs, one at a time, until well incorporated.

Blend in flour, vinegar, and baking soda until incorporated and then transfer the batter into the loaf pan lined with parchment sheet and bake for 30 to 40 minutes or until the bread has cooked and an inserted skewer into the bread slides out clean.

Let the bread cool in the pan, then take it out, cut into ten slices and serve.

Nutrition: 151 cal; 14 g fats; 5 g protein; 3 g net carb; 4 g fiber;

Strawberry Bread

Preparation time: 10 minutes

Cooking time: 15 minutes

Serving: 10

Ingredients

3/4 cup fresh strawberries, chopped

12 tablespoons coconut flour

1/2 teaspoon salt

1 1/2 teaspoon baking powder

1/2 teaspoon cinnamon

1 1/2 teaspoon vanilla extract, unsweetened

5 eggs, pastured

8 tablespoons melted butter, unsalted

1 egg white, pastured

1 cup erythritol sweetener

2 tablespoons whipping cream, grass-fed, full-fat

2 tablespoons sour cream, full-fat

For the icing:

1/4 cup fresh strawberries, chopped

1 tablespoon butter, melted, unsalted

3/4 cup erythritol sweetener

2 tablespoons heavy whipping cream, grass-fed

Directions

Switch on the oven, set it to 350 degrees f and let preheat.

Meanwhile, add eggs and egg whites into a bowl, add sour cream, whipping cream, sweetener, salt, baking powder, vanilla, and cinnamon and beat until combined.

Blend in butter until combined, slowly stir in flour and fold in berries until combined.

Take a loaf pan, line it with parchment paper, pour in batter and bake the cake for 1 hour and 10 minutes or until the bread has cooked and an inserted skewer into the bread slides out clean.

Meanwhile, prepare the icing and for this, place all the ingredients in a bowl, whisk until well combined and set aside. When the bread has baked, let the bread cool in the pan, then take it out, spread the icing on top, cut into ten slices and serve.

Nutrition: 192 cal; 16 g fats; 4 g protein; 3 g net carb; 3 g fiber;

Nut And Seed Bread

Preparation time: 10 minutes

Cooking time: 15 minutes

Serving: 16

Ingredients

1/2 cup flax seed

1/2 cup sesame seeds

1/2 cup pistachios

1/2 cup almonds

1/2 cup cashews

1/2 cup walnuts

1/3 tsp salt

1/4 cup avocado oil

3 eggs, pastured

Directions

Switch on the oven, set it to 325 degrees f and let preheat.

Meanwhile, place all the ingredients in a bowl, and stir until well combined and incorporated.

Pour the batter in a loaf pan, greased with oil, and then bake the bread for 45 minutes or until bread has cooked. Let the bread cool in its pan for 10 minutes, then take it out, transfer it to a wire rack to cool completely, then cut into 12 slices and serve.

Nutrition: 191 cal; 16 g fats; 5 g protein; 3 g net carb; 3 g fiber;

Chocolate Chip Ricotta Bread

Preparation time: 10 minutes

Cooking time: 15 minutes

Serving: 18

Ingredients

1 1/2 cups almond flour, blanched

4 medium bananas, mashed

2 teaspoons baking powder

1 cup ricotta cheese, full-fat

1 cup chocolate chips, unsweetened

2 eggs, pastured

2 teaspoons vanilla extract, unsweetened

Directions

Switch on the oven, set it to 350 degrees f and let preheat.

Meanwhile, place the mashed banana in a bowl, beat in vanilla, eggs, and cheese until combined and then beat in flour, salt, and baking powder until incorporated.

Fold in chocolate chips, pour the mixture into a 9 by 5 inches loaf pan, lined with parchment sheet and bake the bread for 40 to 50 minutes or until the bread has cooked and an inserted toothpick into the bread comes out clean.

Let the bread cool in the pan, then take it out, cut into 18 slices, and serve.

Nutrition: 121 cal; 9.8 g fats; 4.6 g protein; 2 g net carb; 2.2 g fiber;

Butternut Squash Banana Bread

Preparation time: 10 minutes

Cooking time: 15 minutes

Serving: 10

Ingredients

1 3/4 cups almond flour, blanched

1 1/4 cup erythritol sweetener

2 tablespoons coconut flour

1/2 teaspoon salt

1 tablespoon and 1 teaspoon pumpkin pie spice

4 ounces cream cheese, softened

1/2 teaspoon vanilla extract, unsweetened

1/4 cup butter, unsalted, softened

2 eggs, pastured

1 cup pumpkin puree

For the frosting:

1/2 teaspoon cinnamon

1/2 teaspoon vanilla extract, unsweetened

1/2 cup erythritol sweetener

4 ounces cream cheese, full-fat, softened

2 tablespoons butter, unsalted

Directions

Switch on the oven, set it to 350 degrees f and let preheat.

Meanwhile, place cream cheese in a bowl, add butter and sweetener, beat until creamy, beat in eggs, one at a time, and then beat in pumpkin puree and vanilla until mixed.

Stir together flours, salt and pumpkin pie spice in a bowl, slowly stir into the egg mixture until smooth and incorporated and then pour into a greased 9 by 5 inches loaf pan.

Bake the bread for 45 minutes until the bread has cooked and an inserted skewer into the bread comes out clean.

Meanwhile, prepare the frosting and for this, beat together cream cheese and butter until creamy, then beat in cinnamon and vanilla, stir in sweetener and set aside until required.

When the bread has baked, let the bread cool for 10 minutes, then take it out, and transfer the bread on a wire rack to cool completely.

Spread the frosting on the bread, then cut into ten slices and serve.

Nutrition: 173

Cal; 13 g

Fats; 6 g

Protein; 2.3 g

Net carb; 1.3 g

Fiber;

Cranberry Orange Bread

Preparation time: 10 minutes

Cooking time: 15 minutes

Serving: 12

Ingredients

1 cup chopped fresh cranberries

9 tablespoons coconut flour

1 1/2 teaspoon baking powder

3 tablespoons monk fruit powder

1/4 teaspoon salt

9 tablespoons butter, unsalted, melted

1 teaspoon vanilla extract, unsweetened

2/3 cup erythritol sweetener

1 1/2 teaspoon orange extract, unsweetened

5 eggs, pastured

1 egg yolk, pastured

2 tablespoons sour cream

For the glaze:

2 tablespoons monk fruit powder

1/2 tablespoon butter, unsalted, melted

1 teaspoon heavy whipping cream, grass-fed, full-fat

Directions

Switch on the oven, set it to 350 degrees f and let preheat.

Meanwhile, add eggs and egg yolks in a bowl and beat in erythritol, vanilla, butter, sour cream, and orange extract until combined and then beat in flour, salt, and baking powder until incorporated.

Stir together cranberries and 3 tablespoons monk fruit powder until coated, then fold into the prepared batter and pour into a loaf pan lined with parchment paper.

Bake the bread for 50 to 55 minutes or until the bread has cooked and an inserted skewer into the bread slides out clean.

Meanwhile, prepare the glaze and for this, beat together butter, monk fruit sweetener, and cream until mixture reach to the consistency of thick glaze, set aside until required.

When the bread has cooked, top it with prepared glaze, let the bread cool for 15 minutes, then cut into 12 slices and serve.

Nutrition:

139 cal;

12 g fats;

3 g protein;

2 g net carb;

2 g fiber;

Chapter 10.   Special Occasion Recipes

Bread With Beef And Peanuts

Preparation time: 3 hours

Cooking time: 15 minutes

Servings: 8

Ingredients

☐ 15 oz beef meat

☐ 5 oz herbs de provence

☐ 2 big onions

☐ 2 cloves chopped garlic

☐ 1 cup of milk

☐ 20 oz almond flour

☐ 10 oz rye flour

☐ 3 teaspoons dry yeast

☐ 1 egg

☐ 3 tablespoons sunflower oil

☐ 1 tablespoon sugar

☐ sea salt

☐ ground black pepper

☐ red pepper

Directions

1. sprinkle the beef meat with the herbs de provence, salt, black, and red pepper and marinate in bear for overnight.

2. cube the beef and fry in a skillet or a wok on medium heat until soft (for around 20 minutes).

3. chop the onions and garlic and then fry them until clear and caramelized.

4. combine all the ingredients except for the beef and then mix well.

5. combine the beef pieces and the dough and mix in the bread machine.

6. close the lid and turn the bread machine on the basic program.

7. bake the bread until the medium crust and after the bread is ready take it out and leave for 1 hour covered with the towel and only then you can slice the bread.

Nutrition:

Carbohydrates 4 g

Fats 42 g

Protein 27 g

Calories 369

Basic Sweet Yeast Bread

Preparation time: 3 hours

Cooking time: 25 minutes

Servings: 8

Ingredients

☐ 1 egg

☐ ¼ cup butter

☐ 1/3 cup sugar

☐ 1 cup milk

☐ ½ teaspoon salt

☐ 4 cups almond flour

☐ 1 tablespoon active dry yeast

After beeping:

☐ fruits/ground nuts

Directions

1. add all of the ingredients to your bread machine, carefully following the instructions of the manufacturer (except fruits/ground nuts).

2. set the program of your bread machine to basic/sweet and set crust type to light or medium.

3. press start.

4. once the machine beeps, add fruits/ground nuts.

5. wait until the cycle completes.

6. once the loaf is ready, take the bucket out and let the loaf cool for 5 minutes.

7. gently shake the bucket to remove loaf.

8. transfer to a cooling rack, slice and serve.

9. enjoy!

Nutrition: Carbohydrates 2.7 g Fats 7.6 g Protein 8.8 g Calories 338

Apricot Prune Bread

Preparation time: 3 hours

Cooking time: 1 hour

Servings: 8

Ingredients

☐ 1 egg

☐ 4/5 cup whole milk

☐ ¼ cup apricot juice

☐ ¼ cup butter

☐ 1/5 cup sugar

☐ 4 cups almond flour

☐ 1 tablespoon instant yeast

☐ ¼ teaspoon salt

☐ 5/8 cup prunes, chopped

☐ 5/8 cup dried apricots, chopped

Directions

1.add all of the ingredients to your bread machine, carefully following the instructions of the manufacturer (except apricots and prunes).

2.set the program of your bread machine to basic/sweet and set crust type to light or medium.

3.press start.

4.once the machine beeps, add apricots and prunes.

5.wait until the cycle completes.

6.once the loaf is ready, take the bucket out and let the loaf cool for 5 minutes.

7.gently shake the bucket to remove loaf.

8.transfer to a cooling rack, slice and serve.

9.enjoy!

Nutrition:

Carbohydrates 4 g

Fats 8.2 g

Protein 9 g

Calories 364

Citrus Bread

Preparation time: 3 hours

Cooking time: 1 hour

Servings: 8

Ingredients

☐ 1 egg

☐ 3 tablespoons butter

☐ 1/3 cup sugar

☐ 1 tablespoon vanilla sugar

☐ ½ cup orange juice

☐ 2/3 cup milk

☐ 1 teaspoon salt

☐ 4 cup almond flour

☐ 1 tablespoon instant yeast

☐ ¼ cup candied oranges

☐ ¼ cup candied lemon

☐ 2 teaspoons lemon zest

☐ ¼ cup almond, chopped

Directions

1.add all of the ingredients to your bread machine, carefully following the instructions of the manufacturer (except candied fruits, zest, and almond).

2.set the program of your bread machine to basic/sweet and set crust type to light or medium.

3.press start.

4.once the machine beeps, add candied fruits, lemon zest, and chopped almonds.

5.wait until the cycle completes.

6.once the loaf is ready, take the bucket out and let the loaf cool for 5 minutes.

7.gently shake the bucket to remove loaf.

8.transfer to a cooling rack, slice and serve.

9.enjoy!

Nutrition:

Carbohydrates 4 g

Fats 9.1 g

Protein 9.8 g

Calories 404

Fruit Bread

Preparation time: 3 hours

Cooking time: 2 hours

Servings: 8

Ingredients

☐ 1 egg

☐ 1 cup milk

☐ 2 tablespoons rum

☐ ¼ cup butter

☐ ¼ cup brown sugar

☐ 4 cups almond flour

☐ 1 tablespoon instant yeast

☐ 1 teaspoon salt

Fruits:

☐ ¼ cups dried apricots, coarsely chopped

☐ ¼ cups prunes, coarsely chopped

☐ ¼ cups candied cherry, pitted

☐ ½ cups seedless raisins

☐ ¼ cup almonds, chopped

Directions

Add all of the ingredients to your bread machine, carefully following the instructions of the manufacturer (except fruits).

Set the program of your bread machine to basic/sweet and set crust type to light or medium.

Press start.

Once the machine beeps, add fruits.

Wait until the cycle completes.

Once the loaf is ready, take the bucket out and let the loaf cool for 5 minutes.

Gently shake the bucket to remove loaf.

Transfer to a cooling rack, slice and serve.

Enjoy!

Nutrition:

Carbohydrates 5 g

Fats 10.9 g

Protein 10.8 g

Calories 441

Marzipan Cherry Bread

Preparation time: 3 hours

Cooking time: 1 hour

Servings: 8

Ingredients

☐ 1 egg

☐ ¾ cup milk

☐ 1 tablespoon almond liqueur

☐ 4 tablespoons orange juice

☐ ½ cup ground almonds

☐ ¼ cup butter

☐ 1/3 cup sugar

☐ 4 cups almond flour

☐ 1 tablespoon instant yeast

☐ 1 teaspoon salt

☐ ½ cup marzipan

☐ ½ cup dried cherries, pitted

Directions

Add all of the ingredients to your bread machine, carefully following the instructions of the manufacturer (except marzipan and cherry).

Set the program of your bread machine to basic/sweet and set crust type to light or medium.

Press start.

Once the machine beeps, add marzipan and cherry.

Wait until the cycle completes.

Once the loaf is ready, take the bucket out and let the loaf cool for 5 minutes.

Gently shake the bucket to remove loaf.

Transfer to a cooling rack, slice and serve.

Enjoy!

Nutrition:

Carbohydrates 2 g

Fats 16.4 g

Protein 12.2 g

Calories 511

Ginger Prune Bread

Preparation time: 3 hours

Cooking time: 2 hours

Servings: 8

Ingredients

- [ ] 2 eggs

- [ ] 1 cup milk

- [ ] ¼ cup butter

- [ ] ¼ cup sugar

- [ ] 4 cups almond flour

- [ ] 1 tablespoon instant yeast

- [ ] 1 teaspoon salt

- [ ] 1 cup prunes, coarsely chopped

- [ ] 1 tablespoon fresh ginger, grated

Directions

Add all of the ingredients to your bread machine, carefully following the instructions of the manufacturer (except ginger and prunes).

Set the program of your bread machine to basic/sweet and set crust type to light or medium.

Press start.

Once the machine beeps, add ginger and prunes.

Wait until the cycle completes.

Once the loaf is ready, take the bucket out and let the loaf cool for 5 minutes.

Gently shake the bucket to remove loaf.

Transfer to a cooling rack, slice and serve.

Enjoy!

Nutrition: Carbohydrates 4 g Fats 8.3 g Protein 10.1 g Calories 387

Marzipan Bread

Preparation time: 2 hours 10 minutes

Cooking time: 45 minutes

Servings: 8

Ingredients

☐ 4 eggs

☐ ½ cup butter

☐ ¾ cup sugar

☐ 1 tablespoon vanilla sugar

☐ 2 ½ cups almond flour

☐ 1 tablespoon baking powder

☐ ¼ cup almond, ground

☐ ½ cup marzipan, grated

Directions

Add all of the ingredients to your bread machine, carefully following the instructions of the manufacturer (except marzipan).

Set the program of your bread machine to cake/sweet and set crust type to light.

Press start.

Once the machine beeps, add marzipan.

Wait until the cycle completes.

Once the loaf is ready, take the bucket out and let the loaf cool for 5 minutes.

Gently shake the bucket to remove loaf.

Transfer to a cooling rack, slice and serve.

Enjoy!

Nutrition:

Carbohydrates 3 g

Fats 18.6 g

Protein 8.7 g

Calories 425

Lemon Fruit Bread

Preparation time: 3 hours

Cooking time: 1 hour

Servings: 8

Ingredients

☐ 1 egg

☐ 1 cup milk

☐ ¼ cup butter

☐ 1/3 cup sugar

☐ 4 cups almond flour

☐ 1 tablespoon instant yeast

☐ 1 teaspoon salt

☐ ½ cup candied lemons

☐ 1½ teaspoon lemon zest, grated

☐ ½ cup raisins

☐ ½ cup cashew nuts

Directions

Add all of the ingredients to your bread machine, carefully following the instructions of the manufacturer (except fruits, zest, and nuts).

Set the program of your bread machine to basic/sweet and set crust type to light or medium.

Press start.

Once the machine beeps, add fruits, zest, and nuts.

Wait until the cycle completes.

Once the loaf is ready, take the bucket out and let the loaf cool for 5 minutes.

Gently shake the bucket to remove loaf.

Transfer to a cooling rack, slice and serve.

Enjoy!

Nutrition:

Carbohydrates 3.9 g

Fats 10.6 g

Protein 10 g Calories 438 Total fat 10.6 g,

Chapter 11.   Bonus Recipes

Vanilla Pecan Cookies

Preparation time: 10 minutes

Cooking time: 20 minutes

Servings: 16

Ingredients:

2 cups of almond flour

2 tbsp of erythritol

½ tsp of baking powder

4 oz of unsalted butter

1 egg

1 tsp vanilla essence

2 tbsp sugar-free maple syrup

16 pecan halves

Directions:

Start by preheating the oven to 320 degrees f and layer a cookie sheet with parchment sheet.

Add almond flour, butter, baking powder, and natvia to a food processor.

Blend well then add vanilla, sugar-free maple syrup, and egg.

Beat again to combine then knead the dough on a floured surface.

Divide the prepared dough into 16 small pieces and roll them into balls.

Place the balls on a cookie sheet and press them down gently.

Press a pecan half at the center of each cookie.

Bake them for 20 minutes approximately.

Serve fresh.

Nutrition:

Calories 114

Total fat 9.6 g

Saturated fat 4.5 g

Cholesterol 10 mg

Sodium 155 mg

Total carbs 3.1 g

Sugar 1.4 g

Fiber 1.5 g

Protein 3.5 g

Coconut Wafer Cookies

Preparation time: 10 minutes

Cooking time: 29 minutes

Servings: 8

Ingredients:

3 large egg whites

3.5 oz coconut, shredded

1/4 cup erythritol

12 drops liquid stevia

1 pinch salt

3 tbsp butter, melted

Directions:

Start by preheating the oven to 300 degrees f.

Add egg whites, salt, stevia, erythritol, and coconut to a bowl.

After mixing them well, add melted butter and mix again.

Drop the dough spoon by spoon on a cookie sheet and press down gently.

Bake for 29 minutes then flip the wafers.

Bake for another 5 minutes. Serve.

Nutrition: Calories 77.8 Total fat 7.13 g Saturated fat 4.5 g

Cholesterol 15 mg   Sodium 15 mg   Total carbs 0.8 g   Sugar 0.2 g   Fiber 0.3 g Protein 2.3 g

Tartar Snickerdoodle Cookies

Preparation time: 10 minutes

Cooking time: 12 minutes

Servings: 8

Ingredients:

3/4 cup almond meal

1 tbsp cream of tartar

2 tsp baking powder

2 tbsp cinnamon, ground

1/2 cup natvia

14 oz of walnut butter

3 eggs

1 tbsp of natvia icing mix, for coating

2 tsp cinnamon, ground, for coating

Directions:

Start by preheating the oven to 350 degrees f.

Take a bowl and add almond meal, baking powder, natvia, cinnamon, and cream of tartar.

Mix well then add eggs and walnut butter.

After mixing it well, add eggs and make a smooth dough.

In a separate bowl, mix natvia icing mix with 2 teaspoons cinnamon.

Take a scoop of the prepared dough and roll into a ball repeating until all dough is used.

Place the balls on the baking sheet and flatten them into cookies.

Sprinkle cinnamon mixture on top.

Bake for approximately 12 minutes.

Serve.

Nutrition:

Calories 288

Total fat 25.3 g

Saturated fat 6.7 g

Cholesterol 23 mg

Sodium 74 mg

Total carbs 9.6 g

Sugar 0.1 g

Fiber 3.8 g

Protein 7.6 g

Peanut Butter Cookies

Preparation time: 10 minutes

Cooking time: 18 minutes

Servings: 6

Ingredients:

12 oz of natural peanut butter

1.5 oz shredded coconut

1/2 cup of xylitol

2 large eggs

1 tsp of vanilla extract

Directions:

Start by preheating the oven to 320 degrees f. Layer a cookie tray with parchment paper.

Put all the ingredients in a mixing bowl and stir well.

Divide the dough into cookies and place them on the cookie sheet.

Bake the cookies for 18 minutes or until golden brown.

Serve.

Nutrition:

Calories 198 Total fat 19.2 g

Saturated fat 11.5 g   Cholesterol 123 mg

Sodium 142 mg   Total carbs 4.5 g   Sugar 3.3 g   Fiber 0.3 g Protein 3.4 g

Sour Cream Cookies

Preparation time: 10 minutes

Cooking time: 11 minutes

Servings: 6

Ingredients:

1 ½ cups almond flour

¼ tsp salt

1 tbsp baking powder

½ tsp garlic powder

½ tsp onion powder

2 large eggs

1/2 cup sour cream

4 tbsp unsalted butter melted

1/2 cup shredded cheddar cheese

Directions:

Start by preheating the oven to 450 degrees f and grease a muffin tray with cooking spray.

Whisk almond flour with garlic powder, onion powder, salt, and baking powder in a large bowl.

In a separate bowl, beat eggs with butter and sour cream until smooth.

Stir in the dry mixture and mix until combined.

Add cheese and divide the batter into the muffin tray evenly.

Bake biscuits for 11 minutes until golden brown on the top.

Serve.

Nutrition: Calories 215 Total fat 20 g Saturated fat 7 g

Cholesterol 38 mg   Sodium 12 mg   Total carbs 8 g   Sugar 1 g   Fiber 6 g Protein 5 g

Chocolate Vanilla Cookies

Preparation time: 10 minutes

Cooking time: 9 minutes

Servings: 8

Ingredients:

¼ cup butter, melted

4 tbsp white erythritol

2 tbsp pure brown erythritol

¾ cup finely ground almond flour

1 egg

½ cup sugar-free chocolate chips

½ tsp sugar-free vanilla extract

½ tsp xanthan gum or guar gum

1 pinch salt

Directions:

Start by preheating the oven to 350 degrees f.

Now, melt the butter in a medium-sized bowl in a microwave for 30 seconds.

Stir in vanilla extract and erythritol then beat well using an egg beater.

Now, add egg and whisk again to combine.

Add the xanthan or guar gum, salt, and almond flour then mix to make a smooth dough.

Fold in chocolate chips and divide the dough into 8 equal-sized balls.

Place them on a cookie tray and flatten them with the back of a spoon.

Bake the cookies for 9 minutes, approximately.

Serve.

Nutrition:

Calories 285

Total fat 17.3 g

Saturated fat 4.5 g

Cholesterol 175 mg

Sodium 165 mg

Total carbs 3.5 g

Sugar 0.4 g

Fiber 0.9 g

Protein 7.2 g

Soft Cream Cheese Cookies

Preparation time: 10 minutes

Cooking time: 15 minutes

Servings: 14

Ingredients:

4 tbsp butter

3/4 cup sweetener

3 oz cream cheese

1 tsp vanilla

1 egg

3 cups almond flour

Directions:

Start by preheating the oven to 350 degrees f.

Layer a cookies sheet with a silicone mat and set it aside.

Beat butter with sweetener in a mixing bowl using a hand mixer.

Stir in cream cheese, vanilla, and egg.

Beat well and add almond flour. Mix until it forms a smooth cookie dough. Divide the dough into 14 cookies and place them on the cookie sheet. Bake the cookies for 15 minutes until golden brown on the top. Serve.

Nutrition: Calories 175 Total fat 16 g Saturated fat 2.1 g Cholesterol 124 mg Sodium 8 mg

Total carbs 2.8 g Sugar 1.8 g Fiber 0.4 g Protein 9 g

Dark Chocolate Cookies

Preparation time: 20 minutes

Cooking time: 5 minutes

Servings: 8

Ingredients:

1/2 cup butter softened

1/3 cup swerve

1 tsp pure vanilla extract

1/2 tsp kosher salt

2 cup almond flour

9 oz dark chocolate chips

8 oz sugar-free chocolate chips

Directions:

Start by beating the butter in a bowl using a hand mixer until fluffy. Stir in salt, vanilla, and swerve then mix until combined. Add almond flour. Mix well to make a dough. Cover this cookie dough with plastic wrap and refrigerate for 15 minutes. Divide the dough into 1-inch balls and flatten them into cookies. Place those cookies on a baking sheet layered with parchment paper.

Melt all the chocolate in a bowl in the microwave for 30 seconds. Stir well and dip the biscuits in the chocolate. Place them on the cookie sheet again and freeze for 5 minutes. Serve fresh.

Nutrition: Calories 167 Total fat 5.1 g Saturated fat 1.1 g

Cholesterol 121 mg Sodium 48 mg Total carbs 8.9 g Sugar 3.8 g Fiber 2.1 g Protein 6.3 g

Lemon Cookies

Preparation time: 10 minutes

Cooking time: 10 minutes

Servings: 9

Ingredients:

1/2 cup unsalted grass-fed butter

1 1/2 tbsp fresh lemon juice

1 1/2 tsp lemon zest

1 tsp vanilla extract

1/3 cup powdered monk fruit sweetener

1 cup + 2 tbsp almond flour

Glaze:

1/3 cup powdered monk fruit sweetener - 2-3 tsp almond milk

Directions: Start by preheating the oven to 350 degrees f and layer a baking sheet with parchment paper. Beat the butter with lemon juice and lemon zest in an electric mixer until creamy. Stir in vanilla, almond flour and monk fruit then mix well until combined. Divide the dough into 9 balls and spread them into cookies. Place the cookies on the baking sheet and bake them for 10 minutes approximately. Meanwhile, prepare the glaze by mixing the sweetener with milk. Drizzle it over the baked cookies. Serve.

Nutrition: Calories 236 Total fat 13.5 g Saturated fat 4.2 g Cholesterol 541 mg

Sodium 21 mg Total carbs 7.6 g Sugar 1.4 g Fiber 3.8 g Protein 4.3 g

3-Ingredient Biscuits

Preparation time: 10 minutes

Cooking time: 12 minutes

Servings: 10

Ingredients:

6 oz almond butter

1 large egg

Erythritol, to taste

½ tsp pure stevia

Directions:

Start by preheating the oven to 350 degrees f.

Beat almond butter in a bowl then whisk in the egg.

Stir in stevia and erythritol. Mix until well combined.

Divide the dough into 10 balls and spread them into cookies.

Place them on a cookie sheet lined with parchment paper.

Bake them for 12 minutes until golden.

Serve.

Nutrition:

Calories 174   Total fat 12.3 g   Saturated fat 4.8 g   Cholesterol 32 mg   Sodium 597 mg

Total carbs 4.5 g   Fiber 0.6 g   Sugar 1.9 g   Protein 12 g

Flaked Almond Biscuits

Preparation time: 10 minutes

Cooking time: 24 minutes

Servings: 8

Ingredients:

1 cup almond meal

1 cup desiccated coconut unsweetened

1 cup flaked almonds

3 1/2 tbsp butter

1/3 cup xylitol

1 tsp vanilla extract

1 tsp baking powder

1 tsp water

2 eggs

Directions:

Start by preheating the oven to 320 degrees f and layer two cookie trays with parchment paper.

Pour almond meal in a large mixing bowl.

Stir in coconut, almonds, or other nuts.

Mix well to combine and set this mixture aside.

Melt butter in a saucepan then add vanilla and xylitol.

Cook for 7 minutes until it turns golden brown.

Remove it from the heat then add water and baking powder.

Mix well then add the remaining dry ingredients and eggs.

Stir until well combined then divide the dough into a tablespoon-sized balls.

Place them on the cookie trays and flatten them using a spoon.

Bake those cookies for 17 minutes until golden brown.

Garnish as desired.

Serve fresh.

Nutrition:

Calories 121

Total fat 12.9 g

Saturated fat 5.1 g

Cholesterol 17 mg

Sodium 28 mg

Total carbs 8.1 g

Sugar 1.8 g

Fiber 0.4 g

Protein 5.4 g

Pecan Snowball Cookies

Preparation time: 40 minutes

Cooking time: 15 minutes

Servings: 24

Ingredients:

8 tbsp ghee

1 1/2 cup almond flour

1 cup pecans, chopped

1/2 cup swerve sweetener

1 tsp vanilla extract

1/2 tsp vanilla liquid stevia

1/4 tsp salt

Powdered swerve, to coat

Directions:

Start by preheating the oven to 350 degrees f.

Throw all the ingredients into a food processor then blend until smooth.

Divide the dough into 24 cookies and roll them in powdered swerve.

Place them on the baking sheet. First, freeze them for 30 minutes in the freezer. Bake them for 15 minutes or until golden brown. Serve.

Nutrition: Calories 190   Total fat 17.5 g   Saturated fat 7.1 g   Cholesterol 20 mg

Sodium 28 mg   Total carbs 5.5 g   Sugar 2.8 g   Fiber 3.8 g Protein 3 g

Chocolate Pecan Cookies

Preparation time: 10 minutes

Cooking time: 12 minutes

Servings: 8

Ingredients:

1 ½ cups powdered swerve

6 tbsp unsweetened cocoa powder

¼ tsp salt

½ cup dark chocolate chips

½ cup chopped pecans

3-4 large egg whites

1 tsp vanilla extract

Directions:

Start by preheating the oven to 350 degrees f.

Layer a baking sheet with parchment paper then spray with cooking oil.

Whisk swerve, pecan, chocolate chips, cocoa, salt, vanilla, and egg whites in a bowl until smooth.

Form the dough into 2-inch cookies.

Place them on the baking sheet and bake them for 12 minutes. Serve.

Nutrition: Calories 237   Total fat 22 g   Saturated fat 9 g   Cholesterol 35 mg   Sodium 118 mg

Total carbs 5 g   Sugar 1 g   Fiber 2 g Protein 5 g

Cookie Sandwiches

Preparation time: 10 minutes

Cooking time: 12 minutes

Servings: 8

Ingredients:

2 1/4 cups almond flour

3 tbsp coconut flour

4 tbsp cocoa powder

1 tsp baking powder

1/2 tsp xanthan gum

1/4 tsp salt

1/2 cup butter, softened

1/2 cup swerve sweetener

1 egg

1 tsp vanilla extract

Cream filling

4 oz cream cheese, softened

2 tbsp butter

1/2 tsp vanilla extract

1/2 cup powdered swerve

Directions:

Start by preheating the oven to 350 degrees f.

Place all the dry ingredients in a mixing bowl and mix well.

Beat butter with swerve for 2 minutes until fluffy.

Stir in vanilla and egg until combined.

Whisk in the dry mixture then mix well to form the dough.

Divide this dough into two parts and spread each part into a 1/8-inch sheet.

Use a cookie cutter to neatly cut the cookies out of these sheets.

Place them on a cookie sheet and bake for 12 minutes approximately.

Meanwhile, prepare the filling by beating butter with cream cheese and vanilla extract in a bowl.

Once baked, place half of the cookies on a cookie sheet.

Top them with the prepared filling.

Place the remaining baked cookies on top of the filling.

Serve.

Nutrition:

Calories 331

Total fat 12.9 g

Saturated fat 6.1 g

Cholesterol 10 mg

Sodium 18 mg   Total carbs 9.1 g   Sugar 2.8 g   Fiber 0.8 g Protein 4.4 g

Red Lobster Biscuits

Preparation time: 10 minutes

Cooking time: 23 minutes

Servings: 8

Ingredients:

2 cups almond flour

2 tsp baking powder

½ tsp garlic powder

½ tsp onion powder

½ tsp kosher salt

1 pinch cracked black pepper

¼ cup green onions, finely sliced

2 eggs, beaten

½ cup grass-fed butter, melted

½ cup cheddar cheese, shredded

Directions:

Start by preheating the oven to 350 degrees f.

Pour 2 cups of almond flour in a large bowl.

Add pepper, green onions, garlic powder, onion powder, salt, and baking powder.

Whisk eggs with melted butter in a separate bowl.

Stir in dry mixture and shredded cheese.

Mix well until incorporated then divide the dough into small cookies.

Bake them for 23 minutes in the oven.

Serve.

Nutrition:

Calories 179

Total fat 15.7 g

Saturated fat 8 g

Cholesterol 323mg

Sodium 43 mg

Total carbs 4.8 g

Sugar 3.6 g

Fiber 0.8 g

Protein 5.6 g